DR. ART
HISTER'S

GUIDE TO
LIVING A
LONG &
HEALTHY
LIFE

DR. ART HISTER'S

GUIDE TO
LIVING A LONG & HEALTHY LIFE

Art Hister, M.D.

GREYSTONE BOOKS
Douglas & McIntyre Publishing Group
Vancouver / Toronto / Berkeley

To my fantastic and loving family—Phyllis, Bix, Bucky,
and now including the incredible Vivi

Greystone Books
A division of Douglas & McIntyre Ltd.
2323 Quebec Street, Suite 201
Vancouver, British Columbia
Canada v5T 4S7
www.greystonebooks.com

National Library of Canada Cataloguing in Publication Data
Hister, Art
  Dr. Art Hister's guide to living a long & healthy life / Art Hister
  Includes bibliographical references and index
  ISBN 1-55365-018-2
  1. Self-care, Health. I. Title II. Title: Guide to living a long & healthy life.
RC81.H582 2003   616.02'4   C2003-911239-X

Library of Congress information is available upon request

Editing by Nancy Flight
Copy editing by Pamela Robertson
Cover design by Val Speidel
Cover photograph by Chick Rice
Printed and bound in Canada by Friesens
Printed on acid-free paper
Distributed in the U.S. by Publishers Group West

We gratefully acknowledge the financial support of the Canada Council for the Arts, the British Columbia Arts Council, and the Government of Canada through the Book Publishing Industry Development Program (BPIDP) for our publishing activities.

Contents

Acknowledgments

As always, this effort could never have been completed without a significant amount of help.

This whole project has been nurtured, nudged, and nuzzled by my wonderful publisher, Rob Sanders, who is not only a gentleman of great intelligence (he hired me, after all) but an equally great guy to work with. And best of all, he takes a joke as well as anyone.

I once again owe a big debt for fixing and cutting the text to manageable proportions to my delightful editor, Nancy Flight, who is fast becoming Jewish, I fear, as I force her to deal with terms that a girl from Ohio does not run across too often. A *bei geizunt*, Nancy.

Those who read parts of the text and added their usual cogent comments include Ramona Josephson, Dr. Ray Baker, Dr. Jack Taunton, Dr. John Fleetham, Dr. Doug Clement, Dr. Wolfgang Linden, and Dr. Brad Fritz. Their help was invaluable.

And then there's the fantastic crew at Innovative Fitness, who put up with my complaints and moans and groans (in part because I pay them, I suppose, but hey, even money has its limits) and who are always so upbeat and such a joy to work with. So thank you, guys, for literally making me into a new man. And an especially big thanks to Guy Demong, who thinks he's handsome and witty and charming, as well as a great actor—and I'm in no position to argue with him or else he'll make me do more squats—and who contributed the section on resistance training exercises.

Finally, there's my wife, Phyllis, who is the boss of me, but hey, folks, that's the way I like it. She is a truly amazing woman who knows perfectly when to cajole, when to encourage, when to harass, and when to leave and go to work. She is the sole reason this project got completed, and the major reason I manage to do anything.

Introduction

Men's courses will foreshadow certain ends, to which
if persevered in, they must lead. But if the course be
departed from, the ends will change.
CHARLES DICKENS, *A Christmas Carol*

We're just a bunch of kids with outdated birth certificates.
THEODORE ROOSEVELT

THE IMPETUS for this book began about three years ago on one of my semiannual vacations, during which I indulge myself in my favorite pastimes of eating, drinking, eating, sleeping, eating, eating, and eating. On that trip, my wife and I were accompanied by our good friends Norm and Jeannie. Although Norm is a great traveling companion, he has one habit that is a bit strange: he is completely and utterly unable to pass a weigh scale without putting some coins in and stepping on it. His eyes light up even when he passes a supermarket produce weigh scale, but so far, thank God, he has resisted the temptation to jump on — at least as far as I know.

Anyway, one day Norm and I were standing around in an idle moment in the lovely Italian town of Perugia, the women having done the usual and gone off shopping without the boys. Norm, of course, instantly decided to pleasure himself by sliding some coins into a weigh scale, which quickly revealed (*quelle surprise!*) that he hadn't gained an ounce since the last time he'd weighed himself, about two hours earlier.

This information, however, only whetted his appetite, but instead of weighing himself again, which apparently went against even his loose standards, Norm started in on me, trying to convince me to step on the scale, in loco Normanis, as it were. This was something I hadn't done in ages, partly because I didn't want to be a codependent in Norm's habit, but also because I had an aversion to weigh scales. You see, for as long as I could remember, I had always been slightly chubby (OK, I was pretty fat), but I hid it well, and I didn't want to be reminded of what I was doing. Besides, I figured, if I really did need periodic reminding of something I didn't want to face up to, I always had my wife to help me out.

But given that we had loads of time that day and little to do, I decided to humor Norm for once, and I got on the scale which—to my great surprise—promptly registered 77 kilograms (169 pounds). To my even greater chagrin, it stayed at that stratospheric reading no matter how much I shifted my stance or banged the side of the scale, which put me in an intense state of shock, not just because this was Italy, where scales are supposed to register one's weight in kilos, but also because at 1.68 meters (5 feet 6 inches), I had to suddenly acknowledge that I was schlepping a hell of a lot of excess poundage all over the country.

When we got back to Vancouver, I immediately did what every Jewish man does when he has a problem—I called a specialist to get an estimate. My family doctor, you may be thinking, or perhaps someone who runs a fat farm, or maybe even an endocrinologist to give me some thyroid pills? No, no, and no, I'm afraid. Rather, I consulted my friend Ben, the plastic surgeon—*excuuuuse* me, the cosmetic surgeon.

"You have to help me, Ben," I pleaded. "You have to get rid of this fat I'm carrying."

"And how exactly do you propose I do that?" asked Ben, nonchalantly skimming a magazine.

"Suck it away, of course. *Pleeeeease!*"

"OK," said Ben, putting down the magazine. "Perhaps I will. But first I have to examine you, so take off your clothes." Although I hate getting naked in front of other men (my favorite joke from childhood: patient says to doctor who has just told him to get undressed, "You first, Big Boy"), I acceded to Ben's request, though I refused to doff my undies, not out of a sense of modesty but because I wanted Ben to see my abdominal rolls tumbling over the ridge of the elastic band of my shorts. *When Ben sees that spillover effect*, I thought, *he can't possibly refuse me.*

After a cursory examination that lasted slightly longer than the time most men spend choosing a suit, that is, thirty seconds (including the time I spent undressing), Ben said, "No can do, Art. Get dressed. Go home."

"No can do what?" I exclaimed.

"No liposuction for you," said Ben, in his best imitation of the Soup Nazi. "Get dressed and go home. I have real patients to see."

"No liposuction for me?" I screamed, drawing a loud guffaw from someone in the waiting room. I couldn't believe what I had just heard from Ben, mainly because I had never encountered a plastic surgeon — excuse me, a cosmetic surgeon — who would turn down the chance to make a quick buck.

"Why the hell can't I get liposuction?"

"Because you have no muscles," Ben smirked.

"I'm flunking liposuction because I have no muscles? Who needs muscles? I'm Jewish, Ben, remember? And besides," I wailed, "I'm willing to pay you," figuring that this rash offer wouldn't really cost me much since a tenet of the Hippocratic oath bound Ben to give me a huge discount on whatever he eventually did.

"Look," he said, "if I did what you want me to do, I would just be taking your money for nothing [maybe Ben hadn't heard of Hippocrates] because for liposuction to be meaningful [meaningful? I need a relationship with my fat tissue?], you need muscles first. Even a tiny bit of muscle will do. Get that, and then I'll take your money."

"But where can I get muscles at my age?" I moaned. And that's when sleek, slim Ben proceeded to tell me about his fitness regime and his fitness club.

So the next day found me being interviewed — yes, interviewed, because, Ben had told me pointedly, "They don't take just anybody at my fitness club"—by a Schwarzenegger-type punk younger than either of my sons who had massive biceps and triceps and several other sets of ceps bulging out of his too-tight top and who was oblivious to my protestations that I didn't really need a personal trainer, that I didn't really want to be buff, that all I really wanted was enough muscle to pass liposuction.

Well, the rest, as they say, is history, because after a few sessions at that club, I got hooked on fitness. Yes, hooked: my name is Art, and I'm a fitness junkie because I now visit that same fitness club at least three times a week, and I run on my own two or three more times a week.

But wait, folks, there's more. As part of my newfound health regime, I have also started eating much better than I used to, in large part, I suppose, because my wife became a committed vegetarian (all vegetarians either are—or should be—committed) about the same time I became a fitness fiend, but also in part because I knew that to get healthier, I had to discontinue my ethnically based habit of eating meat, meat, and more meat, not to mention fats, too, at every opportunity. And as a result, I'm much healthier than I was the day Norm goaded me to step on that scale in Perugia.

"Really?" some of you skeptics will no doubt wonder, looking at my picture on the dust jacket. "This guy is healthy? Does he really look healthy to you, Martha?"

Really, George, trust me. I'm healthy, or at least much healthier than I used to be. I'm proud to say that I now weigh about 61 kilograms (135 pounds). Actually, 59.8 kilograms (132.4 pounds) this morning, and yes, of course that's with no clothes on; I mean, what neurotic would ever weigh himself with even one stitch on, eh? And I even managed to get down to 58 kilograms (128 pounds) once, but alas, that only lasted for about three hours because my wife kept telling everyone we ran into who remarked on my new svelte form that I had developed an eating disorder.

I have also twice gone back to weighing more than 62.5 kilograms (140 pounds)—until panic set in and I quickly returned to my goal of weighing in the vicinity of 61. (To learn why I want to weigh around 61 kilograms, you'll have to read the information about BMI in the section on weight.)

But hey, folks, here's the thing: I can now get into pants that I last wore over thirty years ago (never mind asking why I still have thirty-year-old pants; bell-bottoms came back, didn't they, so why not polyester?), and you know what's even more impressive? Some of the weight I now carry is in the form of new—ta da!—muscle. Thus, my waist has gone from size 36 to size 31 (30, if I really, really, really hold my breath and the manufacturer has allowed for a bit of stretching at the beltline), and my biceps (I didn't even know I had biceps until recently) have grown by almost an inch.

But weight redistribution and reduction and new acquaintance with muscle tissue are only two of the benefits my health and fitness regime has given me. I also have way more energy than I had the few years before I started on this road. Plus, I sleep longer and better than I used to, I have much better concentration than I did (at least for things I want to concentrate on, like the name and rank of every Iraqi muckamuck still in hiding in Syria), I have much better aerobic capacity, my sense of self-esteem has risen greatly (though some might argue that it never needed enhancement), and I'm much stronger than I have ever been. And what's perhaps most impressive of all is that I actually look buff. Yes, even sideways, and even when I don't hold my breath.

To underline just how healthy and strong I feel, last summer, I and my equally fit wife (after noting the change in my physique—namely, that I finally had one—my wife adopted the same fitness program) did something we'd postponed for thirty years: we spent six days and nights trekking the West Coast Trail on Vancouver Island, 74 kilometers (46 miles) of wilderness bordering the Pacific Ocean, over which we had to schlep all our own food and gear. And we survived!

So there you have it, folks—the slightly longish version of the main reason I wanted to write this book: to convince you that you can also become healthier and probably live longer, as well. As my kids keep telling everyone who marvels at the new me, "Hey, guys, if this fat old fart can do it, anyone can."

You see, as a health educator, I have reams and reams of studies and statistics showing that the majority of you out there are not paying enough attention to your health. And as a midlife do-gooder (midlifers are far more likely than any other demographic group to get involved in charitable activities, such as writing this book), I feel I have to do my bit to help you change your lives for the better, especially since there is finally some evidence that a few of you—too few, but still, some may be ready to make the appropriate changes.

According to a report entitled *Health Care in Canada 2002*, "more than half of Canadians have taken health into their own hands." On first reading, this information scared the daylights out of me because it sounded as if some of you had started doing your own appendectomies and vasectomies, which would not be a huge surprise given the waits for surgery these days. But on sober reanalysis, I realized this probably meant that a growing number of Canadians are consulting publications and the Internet for health information—in part, I suppose, because you can do that sitting down, and anything that can be done from a sitting position is an easier sell to North Americans than something that requires even a slight effort. Along the same lines, a report from May 2002 found that 72 percent of American adult women and 51 percent of American adult men had surfed the Internet looking for health information, and nearly two-thirds had done so seeking information about exercise, nutrition, and weight control.

On the depressing other hand, however, there are too many of you who still believe—or want to believe—that despite all the evidence to the contrary, lifestyle doesn't really make much of a difference in health matters. These people invariably love to say things like, "For 80 years, you know, my Fat Uncle Jean-Marc (Quebecers are real experts at this) drank one pint of whiskey and smoked two packs of cigarettes every day, eh; he never ate a veggie that wasn't deep-fried or buried in butter or mixed with poutine, eh; *mon oncle*, eh, he never did a lick of exercise, and that Fat Jean-Marc, eh, he lived to a hundred, and he died in his sleep, eh, dreaming of chorizo, confit, and Cold Duck."

"So?"

"So my uncle, God rest his soul, eh, had great genes and hey, he's my uncle, so, eh..."

"You mean he was your uncle."

"Whatever, eh, but hey, I have the same genes."

If only, people, if only. True, genes are important in determining how long you live and also what you are likely to die from; several studies have found that people who live to be centenarians most likely make it that far primarily because of great genes. Indeed, according to some theories, the human body was not designed for long-term use, so even if the average person did all the right things healthwise, she would still be unlikely to add many years to her mortal existence. One expert even claims that if we were able to eliminate all the major diseases—heart disease, cancer, diabetes, and stroke—that currently knock off the majority of us, we'd still only add about fifteen years or so to the average life expectancy.

Why? Because, according to this school of thought, your genes, which are the driving force of evolution, have no interest in you after you cease to be of use to them, so evolution stops caring about you after you have reached geezerhood, when you can no longer pass on your genetic material, or not as easily, anyway. In other words, this argument goes, we are largely captive to our genes, and there is bloody little we can do about it. It's a view that clearly appeals to those of us who don't want to do anything more active than pretaping another episode of *Friends*.

But lots of people—me included—don't agree with that fatalistic view and we point to trends in diseases to back our claims. For example, over the past two decades, the number of North Americans (including, alas, children) with Type 2 diabetes has risen dramatically. The reason for this increase is simple: since our genes have clearly not changed much—if at all—in that short burst of evolutionary time, the only explanation is the concurrent explosion of obesity in our midst, which will eventually result in a far higher incidence of strokes, heart attacks, kidney disease, and premature death at all ages.

And obesity, I'm afraid, is largely a result of lifestyle factors. A study from California's Lawrence Berkeley National Laboratory found that identical twins can end up with much different weights solely because of the choices they make about whether and how much they exercise and what food they eat. The title of the study, by the way, should capture your attention: *Exercise and Not Genetics Is Major Determinant of Weight*.

Swedish scientists studying 50,000 pairs of twins attempted to come up with a number you can rely on—How much of what I have to work with is genetics? How much is my lifestyle?—and concluded that a "maximum of around a third of the variance in longevity is attributable to genetic factors, and almost all of the remaining variance is due to non-shared, individual specific environmental factors." In English, this means that you should do more exercise and eat better because lifestyle factors account for 67 percent of the difference between how long you live and how long your brother lives.

Further, according to a 25-year Scottish study, typical Fat Uncle Jocks—that is, overweight male Scottish smokers—are very likely to die before the age of 70, while thin, lifelong nonsmokers are very likely to live to at least age 70, and many live well beyond that.

Even when you get to a certain age (on instructions from my publisher, I cannot refer to any of you as "old" until later in the book because by then even all you old people will be hooked), lifestyle factors can still make a huge difference in life expectancy. Thus, a study from China found that elderly Chinese who did moderate amounts of exercise (and who never smoked) were less likely to die over the subsequent three years than elderly Chinese who did not exercise regularly.

But even if the depressing theory guys are right that by adopting a healthy lifestyle we can add a maximum of a decade or maybe two to our tab, that's still a pretty significant addition, if you ask me.

I may not be a maths genius (my Cambridge-educated brother-in-law—I think he got a Ph.D. in punting boats down the Thames—swears that the correct word for things to do with numbers is "maths," not "math," and since he has an English accent, he must be right), but two decades on top of six or even seven is still a tremendous amount of time (25 to 33 percent extra, if you do the maths) to add onto your life by living healther.

Just as important, though, a healthy lifestyle is likely to significantly improve the quality of whatever time—short, intermediate, or long—you do have left among us. So even if, as some of you insist, you wouldn't really mind dying young, so long as you could live without paying any attention to what you eat or how active you are, most of you probably would mind very much living a long, impaired (because of chronic illness) life. The chances of that happening when you don't adhere to a healthy lifestyle are rather great these days because we are now much better able to keep you alive with conditions that previously meant a quick death sentence. According to a report from the American Association of Retired Persons (the Jewish chapter is known as the Alte Kackers and Kvetchers Society), a lot more 50-year-old Americans are likely to live to age 80 than was the case just a few short years ago, but most of them will spend their last years suffering from chronic, debilitating conditions that significantly worsen the quality of their daily lives. But here's the thing: most of those conditions can be prevented—or, at the very least, postponed—through healthy lifestyle practices.

Thus, according to an American study carried out over half a century, midlife men who had the healthiest lifestyle habits—the most important being not smoking, using alcohol only moderately, maintaining an appropriate weight, and doing regular exercise—were by far the most likely to end up with a "healthy, happy, and longer life." *Quod erat demonstrandum:* live better and you live better. And longer, too, of course.

So why don't more of you pay attention to your lifestyles? For many, the answer is simple: it's not worth the effort. In a recent survey a majority of Americans polled told the researchers that although "maintaining good physical health" is very important to them, eating well and exercising were "less important objectives." Not to be outdone by their American cowboy cousins, in a British study, nearly 50 percent of Brits said they would rather die a year early than give up smoking, eating the way they do, and drinking alcohol, and in this survey, the young, who of course always figure that they're never going to die, were far more likely to take that view than were midlifers.

Much of this mortal arrogance comes, of course, from the fact that even though we generally acknowledge that we will die one day, most of us somehow expect (or at least hope) that our own demise will be sudden, swift, and free of suffering and pain. Well, yes, that's indeed how some of you will be reintroduced to your maker, but many of you will not die so simply and neatly, or dare I say, quickly. According to current studies, the risk of dying of a sudden, massive terminal heart attack is actually decreasing, and a growing number of you can instead look forward to dying of slowly debilitating heart failure, for example, or cancer, both of which are largely caused by an unhealthy lifestyle. Yes, even cancer. That Swedish study of twins that I cited earlier concluded that "environmental" factors—a European euphemism for lifestyle factors such as smoking, alcohol use, sun exposure, and diet—account for up to 82 percent of the risk of getting cancer.

"Which cancers?" you wonder, as you hurriedly palpate your neck or armpit. The answer is nearly every cancer you can name. U.K. researchers have concluded that the "environment" accounts for 47 percent of thyroid cancers, 75 percent of breast cancers (despite the widespread belief that genes play a larger role in breast cancer than lifestyle does), 74 percent of testicular cancers, 78 percent of cervical cancers, 79 percent of melanomas, 90 percent of lymphomas, and 92 percent of lung cancers. But the balancing good news, folks, is that you can do a lot to alter the Angel of Death's malignant agenda. You just have to make up your mind to do it.

By the way, if, like so many, you're calmly waiting till you get your first symptoms, the robins of disease, before you start to make the appropriate changes to your life, here's something else to munch on. A health research group from Minnesota did a battery of cardiac tests on the first 333 seemingly healthy people who came into their clinic, and they found that—I hope you're not working out on a step machine when you read the next bit because you might fall off and injure yourself—over half of them already had (at the very least) "early" cardiac disease. These people, however, had no idea of their poor states of health, and if they didn't know what their arteries and heart were like, let me ask you: do you know what your cardiovascular system has been up to while you were paying attention to other, more urgent matters? Indeed, you do not, so whether you have symptoms or not, it's really time to get healthy.

And I make an especially strong appeal to parents to start paying more attention to their lifestyles, because there is plenty of evidence that your kids are likely to have the same attitude toward healthy living as you do. Not only that, but if you engage in risky behavior, your kids are much more likely to engage in risky behavior, too, though their idea of taking risks doesn't always align itself with yours. For example, studies show that if parents smoke, kids are more likely to become smokers, as well, but they are also more likely to be sexually active and to drink alcohol at a younger age and to "participate in delinquent behavior."

And another thing: if you think this doesn't apply to you because, well, because you're too old (I am defying my publisher, and besides, this is later in the book), let me tell you, folks, you're never too old and it's never too late to make improvements to your lifestyle. There's always something to gain, no matter how old you are. For example, a recent study found that seniors could significantly lower their risk of a heart attack by adding two slices of whole-grain bread, especially a dark grain, to their daily diet.

One last thing: if you haven't listened to all the health messages you've been inundated with in the past, you may now be wondering what makes me think you will listen to what I have to say. I guess I'm just a terminal optimist (bought Enron at $80, $40, $30, $20, and $1, and I still think it can bounce back) who's always hoping that if the message is delivered to you in a way that hits home, some of you will finally do the maths and start trying to live better. And when you think on it, why would any of you have bought this book if you weren't at least slightly interested in improving your lives?

My main selling point is this: my message is pretty simple. I don't offer you so many choices that you won't be able to decide among them, and I don't overload you with information (if you want to know about the health benefits of royal jelly, for instance, look somewhere else). I also don't promise panaceas for all your ills and troubles. When something doesn't work or isn't true, I say so very clearly, even if it is something my colleagues and I once strongly believed in. And perhaps most important is that I keep fun and pleasure in mind with all my recommendations. Everything I advise is (or can become) a pleasant chore for you; yes, even exercise. Hey, I don't even expect very much from you, so if you don't immediately start running, for example, I can live with that.

I just want to tell you what I've learned about the risks you face if you don't exercise or eat right, what I've done in my own life, and how much that has helped me, in the hopes that you will be motivated to make similar changes. Happily, there is evidence that if you increase someone's awareness of their personal risk or harm, they may decide to change their behavior. So I figure that if I can show you where you fall on the risk scale, and how it's not that hard to change that ranking (honest, it's not), you might at least begin to think of starting an exercise regime or eating healthier.

So sit back, relax, read on, and mull over what you read. Besides, mulling is easy; the harder parts will come when you start getting that itch to actually do something for yourself.

1

Exercise

Move It and Lose It

Fitness has to be fun. If it is not play, there will be no fitness. Play, you see, is the process. Fitness is merely the product.
GEORGE SHEEHAN

O NE DAY a few years ago, as I was getting out of the shower, my son burst in, catching me in all my God-given glory. He stood there for several seconds, mouth agape, looking me up and down, eyes registering intense amazement, and then slowly shook his head and murmured as he left, "You know, Dad, there really is no God," leaving me to ponder where I had gone so wrong. I concluded it was his mother's fault.

Well, that was then and this is now, and my son recently burst in on me again as I was getting out of the shower. This time, however, he merely rooted around for whatever it was he needed, and started to leave.

"So what about God?" I yelled at him.

"You need my help with that?" he retorted, and slammed the door.

I thought about my son's changed response for a while and I decided that the likely reason he reacted with such equanimity to my nakedness the second time is that my appearance had improved so much through the exercise I now do that he no longer feels the need to point out the ravages that a poor lifestyle can lead to.

If I could convince you to make just one change in your life, it would be to become more active. All of us, except perhaps for Lance Armstrong and Marion Jones, could benefit greatly from doing more exercise (and from being more active in our day-to-day activities). This chapter is going to tell you why that is so. My secret hope is that I will make exercise so appealing that even before you get to the end of the chapter, many of you will rush off to the nearest park or track or gym to start working out, and those of you who can't or won't rush off to a gym or park may perhaps be tempted to get off the couch and walk to the corner store instead of driving there. As for those of you who won't be driven to manage even that slight effort, I hope you might at least get up and stretch. Hey, I'm easy. I'll take anything, because you have to start somewhere.

The Number One Reason to Do More Exercise

The number one reason you should do more exercise is not that you will end up looking as good as me (I was strongly informed that this is not likely to induce any of you to start exercising, and I have to believe my wife) but rather that doing more exercise is probably the single health improvement most likely to both extend your life and maximize your quality of life in the time you have left on this mortal coil. Let me rephrase that in boldface: **doing more exercise is the single most important lifestyle adjustment you can make to increase your chances of living longer and to improve the quality of whatever time you have left.**

In short, we have discovered what eluded Ponce de León—the fountain of youth—and it's this: just be more active. Or, to quote Miriam Nelson, the director of the Center for Physical Activity Programs and Policy at Tufts University, "Much of what we consider the aging process is really just a lack of physical activity. Physical activity can halt, reverse, or at least slow many of the factors associated with old age." According to Canadian researchers, in a country where two-thirds of the population is "inactive," if more people would do just a minimal amount of exercise, we could cut the death rate from heart disease by 36 percent, from stroke and diabetes by 20 percent, and from breast cancer by 11 percent—not to mention that we could also significantly cut the death rate from other conditions linked to inactivity, such as osteoporosis and colon cancer.

What Is the Proof That Exercise Matters?
In a decade-long study that looked at major risk factors such as obesity, high blood pressure, and smoking, researchers concluded that "inactivity" was the greatest lifestyle risk to health. This study, by the way, comes from the very serious country of Sweden, so you know they weren't joshing (I mean, these people are so serious that the only Swedish joke of the past decade was the goalie on their Olympic hockey team). Also, according to a report from the World Health Organization, among the countries of the European Union, living a typical sedentary existence has overtaken smoking as the greatest cause of ill health.

But, *bien sur,* it's not just among those bourgeois Europeans that more exercise may be the key to a longer and healthier life. In a study from the good old U.S. of A., Stanford University researchers who followed over 6,000 men for six years determined that their risk of premature death was directly related to their exercise capacity as measured by their ability to work out on a treadmill. As the study subjects' ability to run on a treadmill rose, their subsequent risk of death declined in proportion to that ability; men with the highest exercise capacity were four times less likely to die over the following six years than men with the lowest running ability. That's a hell of a difference in risk of death over a very short period of time, if you ask me.

Taking it one step farther, exercise capacity was a better predictor of how long these men would live than all the other measures that are usually considered pivotal in health outcomes, such as blood pressure levels, cholesterol levels, history of smoking, family history, and body mass index. And taking one more step along the line of uncomfortable conclusions, the authors note that even if a man in this study already had other risk factors for premature heart disease, such as high blood pressure or high cholesterol levels, he was still able to significantly lower his risk of dying prematurely by—ahem! ahem!—starting to exercise.

What are fit men less likely to die of? Practically every condition that eventually kills us. Thus, a Finnish study of 1,300 men with an average age of 52 found that not being in shape significantly increased a man's chances of dying for any reason at all. A recent 10-year study of Welsh men found that those who participated in vigorous exercise such as jogging and swimming were about 50 percent less likely to die prematurely—of any cause—than were those Welsh men who exercised lightly (e.g., singing in the choir after coming home from the coal mine) or moderately (e.g., golfing after working in the mine).

But what about women, some of you may be wondering. Well, as you would no doubt expect, there is absolutely no difference between men and women as far as the benefits of exercise are concerned. In a study of 3,000 healthy women, the results were very similar to those for the Stanford study of 6,000 men. The best predictor of how long these women lived over the subsequent six years was their exercise tolerance on a treadmill; women in the highest quintile of exercise capacity had a mortality rate three times as low as women in the lowest quintile, and as I said earlier, that's a hell of a difference. Also, just as for men, these women's exercise capacity on a treadmill was a better predictor of overall mortality than any other parameter of heart health.

Mixing the sexes, which is always fun but dangerous, another study from Stanford found that runners over the age of 50 (men and women who belonged to a running club—serious runners, in other words) were a smashing three times less likely to die over the 13-year period of the study than nonrunners. Equally important, the women runners postponed age-related disabilities by an amazing nine years longer than their nonrunning sisters. That's nine years, people—nine years longer of living without the pain of osteoarthritis, for example, or nine years longer without the major problems associated with the onset of dementia or the restrictions imposed by strokes and neurodegenerative diseases such as Parkinson's disease, and on and on. Kinda makes you want to leap up and start running, don't it? Well, maybe later. First, read more.

And lest seniors excuse themselves here—"Well, it's probably too late for us octogenarians, eh, Abel?"—let me tell you that the life-protecting effect of exercise accrues to seniors, too. A study presented at the 2003 annual meeting of the American Academy of Neurology determined that over a period of 16 years, those seniors who exercised the most were the most likely to make it to age 90 (and please note: other health practices and nutrition habits—such as going to bingo regularly, and eating prunes—had no bearing on determining which 75-year-olds made it to 90).

Anyway, the bottom line is that your current exercise capacity may be the single best predictor of how long you are going to live from this moment on. So ask yourself: just how far can you run without getting breathless?

Before you get too depressed about the answer, though, know this: it does not take long to achieve the benefits of exercise. In 1966, in the Dallas Bed Rest and Training Study, researchers took five typical students from the University of Texas and put them on strict bed rest for three weeks. After 20 days of this regime, during which they were allowed to do nothing except, I suppose, eat as many ribs as they could manage and watch *The Texas Chainsaw Massacre* over and over, these students experienced a decline in physical health that was similar, the researchers say, to having aged about 30 years. The researchers then put these debilitated students on a moderately intense exercise program, and within several months, the students became as fit, according to the researchers, as "elite" athletes.

"Does that mean," you might ask, "that when you're 20 and living in Texas, it's not very hard to become very fit, Texan-style?" Perhaps, but that's not really what makes this study so interesting. Thirty years later, the researchers recontacted these guys (who were no longer students, of course, because even in Texas, you can't stay in school for 30 years, not even if you star on the varsity football team). As you'd no doubt expect, these ex-students were now typical Good Old Boys, that is, beer-swilling, overweight, rib-and-fried-steak-scarfing total Texans, guys as close to being fit as George Bush is to being elected president of End the Arms Race. Somehow, however, the researchers induced these gents to go on a moderately intense exercise program, and within six months, these guys became so fit that they had managed to "reverse" 100 percent of the loss of aerobic capacity they had experienced since 1966. In other words, at the age of 50-plus, these average middle-aged men were able to get back to being nearly as fit as they had been when they were 20 years old.

Bottom line, folks: it doesn't take long to regain your fitness—or to become fit if you've never been fit in the first place. All it takes is time, will, proper training, and more will.

What Health Problems Might You Prevent by Becoming Fit?

HEART AND BLOOD VESSELS

To understand how exercise produces cardiovascular benefits, you first need to know how the heart and cardiovascular system become damaged, and the theory has changed significantly over the past few years. Scientists used to think that heart attacks occurred solely because cholesterol deposits plugged arteries and narrowed them enough to permit blood clots to form, thus killing the heart tissue fed by those arteries. (In strokes, brain cells would die as a result of "plugged" cerebral arteries.) It's now thought, however, that the process is much more complex. It starts with injuries to the arteries from certain toxins (such as cigarette smoke and oxidized LDL, or low-density lipoproteins, the "bad" cholesterol) and other factors (high blood pressure) that damage the delicate lining of blood vessels. The body responds to that damage by bringing in the troops: all sorts of immune cells that attempt to help the blood vessels heal. This combination of immune cells and toxins (especially that dastardly oxidized LDL) causes the lining of arteries to become inflamed, thus inducing other types of cells to migrate there. Eventually, this process produces chronic thickening of the arterial wall, a pad of plaque consisting of calcium, cholesterol, white blood cells, and so on.

We used to be most concerned about large, hard, "stable" plaques that can narrow arteries up to 80 or 90 percent. We now know, however, that most heart attacks (and strokes) probably occur as a result of ruptures or tears in pliant, "unstable" plaques, which usually don't narrow arteries as much as the harder plaques do but have a softer, more unstable cover that ruptures easily. When a rupture occurs, the body rushes in protective chemicals such as clotting factors and other inflammatory fighters that, alas, lead to a higher risk of clotting and thus a heart attack (or stroke). In soccer, that would be called an "own-goal"—your body's defense actually leads to a worse outcome.

The great news, though, is that exercise significantly reduces the risks of all those problems. Regular exercise leads to lower risks of fatal heart attacks, nonfatal heart attacks, strokes, and cardiovascular events (a medical euphemism for sudden death thought to be primarily the result of a fatal disturbance in heart rhythm, which is generally another manifestation of a damaged cardiovascular system).

Overall, studies estimate that dying from coronary disease is reduced by up to 40 percent in those who are physically fit. That means that at any age, a physically fit person is 40 percent less likely to die from a stroke or heart attack or from sudden death due to a cardiac rhythm disturbance than is his beached, bloated brother. Even if you already have damaged arteries or a sick heart (that is, if you've had a previous heart attack or you have high blood pressure or heart failure), studies have determined that you are still very likely to benefit from doing more exercise. Equally important, first-degree relatives of people who have heart disease can help their own prognoses significantly by doing more exercise.

As for strokes (which, by the way, most stroke experts now call "brain attacks" because they are largely caused by the same factors as heart attacks), exercise significantly lowers the risk of getting, and dying from, a stroke. A study from the famous Cooper Institute in Texas looked at over 16,000 men of varying fitness levels and determined that the most fit men had a 68 percent lower risk of stroke than the least fit men—and the thing is, guys, that even men deemed to be only moderately fit (running 20 to 40 minutes three to five times a week) had nearly the same lowered risk (63 percent) of stroke as did the most fit men.

And although heart disease is often thought of as a "male" disorder, let me stress that cardiovascular disease kills over three times as many women as do all forms of cancer combined—yes, including even breast cancer—so women have at least as much to gain from doing more exercise as do men.

So now let's answer that big question: how does exercise help the cardiovascular system?

To start, regular exercise is an excellent tool for lowering your blood pressure and keeping it at healthy levels. For both men and women, exercise provides better control of blood pressure than any other change in lifestyle, including restricting your salt intake and avoiding alcohol. A recent study concluded that the combination of a low-fat, high-fruit-

and-veggie diet and moderately intense exercise of 180 minutes a week can lower raised blood pressure without requiring the intervention of medication. Exercise also lowers "slightly high" blood pressure (a highly dubious concept, by the way, because after all, "high is high," as my Free Clinic friends used to say, albeit in another context) and "borderline high" blood pressure, and helps those with normal blood pressure maintain their normal levels. It even helps those people who have white coat hypertension, in which one's blood pressure shoots up only in the presence of a scary health professional (especially a doctor, of course).

By the way, as with those new notions about heart attacks, it turns out that the medical profession has also had to alter its views about blood pressure. For nearly two centuries, we've told our patients that the lower register of blood pressure, the diastolic pressure, was the key measure in determining future risks of heart attack and stroke and all those other dreadful things that occur as a result of high blood pressure. Anything over 90 diastolic was cause for concern, though 90 to 100 was considered "borderline" and simply merited careful monitoring. As for the upper register, or systolic pressure, we considered anything over 140 to be "raised," but we also allowed most people, especially the elderly, to get away with raised systolic pressures on the theory that, well, shifts happen, eh? Since systolic pressure rises with age, why worry about it, especially since blood-pressure-lowering medications commonly lead to bothersome side effects and complications?

But my, how times have changed. We now "know" that in most people, the systolic pressure is more important than the diastolic pressure in determining future health risks. As well, we've changed our views on healthy levels of blood pressure. Most experts now believe that any blood pressure reading higher than 120/80 should—at the very least—be monitored regularly, and people with such previously "normal" readings should now be strongly encouraged to modify their lifestyles. In fact, one recent study concluded that people with "high normal" blood pressure (130–139/85–89) may already have early signs of cardiovascular disease, which has led some experts to declare that anyone with a reading between 120/80 and 140/90 is actually suffering from a new health condition called "pre-hypertension."

This realignment of blood pressure levels, by the way, has major implications in the real world. We used to say that about 20 to 25 percent of the population had high blood pressure (most of whom didn't know it), but with these new parameters, up to 50 percent of the population has high blood pressure, and clearly the overwhelming majority still doesn't know it. Even worse, according to most estimates, the large majority of those folks who know about their raised blood pressure do not manage to lower it to what is considered a normal level, and that leads to Problem City. According to a recent estimate, at least 22 percent of heart attacks and 34 percent of strokes in seniors are a direct result of not controlling known high blood pressure well enough.

Exercise also benefits the cardiovascular system by improving lipid levels (lipids are fats), both by lowering LDL levels and by raising those very important HDL levels (HDL stands for high-density lipoprotein, that good-fat guy that rides posse on LDL and sashays it out of the bloodstream and into the liver, where it can be degraded; lots of people now believe that raising HDL probably does more for cardiac health than does lowering LDL).

And as for those couch cantaloupes who would prefer to deal with their cholesterol problems simply by trying to eat better without doing more exercise, I'm afraid it just won't work, guys. Several studies have shown that you are much more likely to achieve your cholesterol goals if you marry an exercise regime to a healthy diet.

Even for all those millions of people who prefer chemical answers to all their health ills and who would much prefer to treat their abnormal cholesterol levels with drugs only, studies have shown that high-risk individuals who combine exercise (and diet) with a statin drug (the most preferred cholesterol-lowering medications) are up to 67 percent less likely to suffer a heart attack than those people who take statins alone. Or to quote Alan Cassel, a drug-policy expert, "The best way to beat heart disease is to take your statin pill for a five-mile walk every morning." Amen.

Exercise also helps the heart by controlling weight, and excess weight is by itself related to much poorer cardiac status. Exercise is especially adept at reducing abdominal fat, or weight around the middle, which is where we tend to put on weight as we age, especially those of us of the male persuasion. When those fat stores are visible, they form what has become known as a "spare tire," leading to what is commonly called an apple shape. (In contrast, people who store fat around the hips or on the thighs or butt have what is known as a pear shape.

Also, fat stores are not always visible, because much abdominal fat is also stored around the viscera (your internal organs), in a form that can only be seen with specialized scans.

No matter where you store it, though, abdominal fat seems to have a particularly malignant effect on your heart and arteries (as well as on your risk of diabetes and some types of cancer, too). In one study of postmenopausal women, abdominal fat raised the risk of premature atherosclerosis (hardening of the arteries) more than overall obesity did (and there is, of course, no reason to believe that this doesn't also hold true in younger women and in men). But here's the thing: the best way to lose weight around the middle—in fact, the only way I know that really works—is to just work it off. Vigorous exercise is an excellent tool for reducing visceral fat in a short period of time. And it's not that hard to do. It takes about 3,500 calories to burn off one pound of fat, and you burn around 100 to 120 calories per mile on an easy run.

Another very important way that regular exercise helps your cardio-vascular system is by keeping your blood vessels young and strong. As you age, your blood vessels, especially your arteries, lose their flexibility and grow harder, and that contributes to a raised risk of heart attacks and strokes, though as many aging men (not to mention their lovers) will concur, some blood vessels actually become much more flexible and softer with age. But then, as at least one female cynic has unkindly pointed out, "Those are not really arteries, guys, more like capillaries." Who says long-time feminists don't have a sense of humor, eh? Hey, she married me, didn't she?

Anyway, exercise helps your blood vessels—arteries as well as capillaries—stay expandable. One study found that the arteries of seniors who exercised were twice as flexible as the arteries of sedentary seniors. In fact, according to the researchers, exercising seniors had arteries that were nearly as expandable as those of people *half their age*, which is either a compliment to the elderly exercisers or a knock on sedentary youngsters. Another study found that previously sedentary, overweight women in their sixties who took up walking for 13 weeks restored the elasticity of their arteries to that of "young women." In fact, the lead researcher declared that this change actually "reversed" the aging process.

And, of course, it's never too late to help your blood vessels. A study showed that people in their nineties who were induced to start moving around their apartments more often developed more pliable arteries than similar nonagenarians who remained inactive. To no surprise, the ones who moved the most had the greatest gain in arterial flexibility.

And then there's inflammation. It is now widely accepted that inflammation plays a key role in heart disease, especially in explaining why some seemingly low-risk individuals suffer heart attacks or strokes. It has always frustrated physicians, you see, not to mention their patients, that many heart attacks and strokes occur in thin, active people and that half of all heart attacks occur in people who have what are considered "normal" cholesterol levels. It's clear that something else exceedingly deleterious must be occurring in these seemingly low-risk people's coronary arteries to result in such major damage, and an important part of that something else is now thought to be inflammation, which might even have its source elsewhere in the body. That's why, for example, we've seen many recent studies that have attempted to link ulcers or even inflamed gums (periodontal disease), to a raised risk of heart disease—a tie my dentist has desperately tried to turn to his advantage with several huge signs in his office declaring Floss or Die. *Pace* my dentist, however, there is no proof as yet that even a lifetime of brushing, flossing, and regular dental check-ups can lead to fewer heart attacks or strokes, though regular dental check-ups certainly do improve your dentist's health—by affording him more vacation time, and a bigger house.

Anyway, exercise is a powerful tool for lowering markers of inflammation such as C-reactive protein, or CRP. And you must remember those initials, folks, because I assure you they will soon rival (perhaps even outrank) "cholesterol" in your cardiovascular vocabulary. According to one study done on 28,000 women, CRP was a better marker for future risk of heart attacks than was LDL. Not that LDL is unimportant. Indeed, in this study, women with high LDL levels were also at greater risk of heart attacks, but the women with the highest risk were those who had high levels of both LDL and CRP.

In men, a recent decades-long study of 8,000 guys from the Honolulu Heart Program concluded that middle-aged men with the highest levels of CRP were four times as likely to eventually have a stroke than were men with the lowest CRP levels. This higher risk of stroke held true even if the men didn't have high blood pressure and diabetes, two major risk factors for stroke. In other words, even seemingly low-risk middle-aged men may be more likely to suffer a stroke if their CRP levels are elevated. And a third recent study found that people with high CRP levels were not able to lower their cholesterol levels through diet nearly as well as those with normal CRP levels.

The good news is that according to a study presented at the annual meeting of the American College of Cardiology in 2003, the more you exercise, the lower your CRP levels. This anti-inflammatory effect can occur in virtually everyone who exercises enough: men and women, young and old, those with established heart disease and those with no signs of active heart disease, the obese and the thin, smokers and non-smokers, those with a high genetic tendency for heart disease and those at seemingly no increased risk—the waterfront, in other words.

Exercise also lowers homocysteine levels. You don't know what homocysteine is? Well, I'll tell you, because hey, you need something else to worry about, don't you? Homocysteine is an amino acid that's a product of protein breakdown, and high homocysteine levels have been linked, particularly in women, to health problems such as heart disease (especially, according to the Framingham Study, heart failure), strokes, even dementia and Alzheimer's disease. For example, another recent study concluded that the higher the homocysteine level in a group of elderly Italians, the poorer their thinking capacities—the really badly off ones had no clue if they were drinking grappa or espresso. Risk factors for higher homocysteine levels include being male (boo!), getting older (boooo!), smoking, high coffee intake (booooooooo!), genes, hypothyroidism, high alcohol intake, and low vitamin-B intake (see chapter 4).

Exercise also reduces the risk of cardiovascular problems by lowering blood levels of proteins and chemicals that boost the blood's tendency to clot, and exercise might even help dissolve blood clots, especially in overweight people, who are at high risk for these potentially lethal problems.

In addition, exercise can be beneficial for those with established heart problems, such as heart failure. Although people with heart failure have traditionally, alas, been told to take it easy so as not to further task their already failing hearts, I'm afraid that this is yet another medical instance of "Oops, we're sorry, but in fact we were wrong." We now know that people with heart failure (as well as those who've already had a heart attack) may be among those who have the most to gain by becoming more active.

Exercise also improves collateral circulation. That is, if your coronary arteries are gradually getting blocked, exercise not only will help keep those arteries open longer (exercise may even enlarge your coronary arteries in the first place) but will also help your body develop new blood vessels that can supplement the work of those partially blocked arteries and help move blood around the blocked areas.

Exercise also improves the beating capacity of the heart and its efficiency, which also lowers your heart rate. Some doctors believe that our hearts have only a limited number of beats in them before they fail, so the slower your heart rate, the better for your heart.

Exercise also lowers stress and anxiety levels (see Chapter 9) and improves mood, and high-stress levels and depression are both related to a raised risk of heart disease. Depression may be particularly damaging to the heart. Studies show that depressed individuals are three to four times more likely to die from heart attacks than are their nondepressed peers, though there is also good evidence that treating depression lowers that risk.

Finally, exercise improves insulin resistance, which lowers the risk of diabetes, and that in turn reduces the risks of heart attack and stroke.

CANCER

This might surprise many of you, but exercise is especially important in preventing cancer. A 25-year study found that the men who were most fit when the study began were about half as likely to die from cancer as the least fit men. The American Cancer Society estimates that 35 percent of cancer deaths can be related to either lack of activity or obesity, and we're not talking about obscure cancers, either.

Breast cancer

A study from the Alberta Cancer Board found that postmenopausal women who reported the greatest amount of activity in their lives were 30 percent less likely to develop breast cancer than were women with the lowest levels of activity. And I have to commend the researchers for being prescient enough to note that housework counts; that is, women who did the most housework over their lifetimes had the lowest risk of developing breast cancer. As a thoughtful and solicitous husband, I instantly pinned this news item to our fridge door (I know my wife knows where the fridge is because we're always running out of juice). She saw the notice, I'm happy to say, though the results were not quite as I imagined, and it took more than two weeks for me to recover. Some people just don't want to be helped, I guess.

Digestive cancers

A study that followed over 7,000 men for 19 years found that men who did more exercise had lower risks of several digestive cancers, such as esophageal cancer, pharyngeal cancer, and stomach cancer. For a separate study, English researchers combed the medical literature and concluded that regular exercise can cut the risk of bowel cancer by up to 50 percent.

Urinary tract cancers

The aforementioned English study also found that exercising men had lower rates of two really low-down cancers, prostate cancer and bladder cancer.

BUT HOW, YOU MAY WONDER, could exercise lower the risk of so many disparate cancers? Well, exercise keeps your weight down, and excess weight, especially abdominal weight, is strongly related to an increased risk of cancer, probably because excess abdominal weight raises the levels of hormones (such as insulin and estrogen), which in turn raises the risk of some cancers. Obese women, for example, have a higher incidence of breast cancer than do normal-weight women. As well, a recent study linked higher insulin levels to a higher risk of dying from nearly all types of cancer.

The only fly in this do-exercise-to-lower-your-risk-of-cancer ointment is that, as any lazy person will quickly point out, "Since cancer takes so long to develop, wouldn't you agree, Art, that exercise works best as a cancer-reducer only if you start exercising early in life? So it's too late for me, eh?"

Well, my friend, you may be partly right. Girls who take up exercise at a young age and continue to do it throughout life are probably lowering their risk of breast cancer much more than seniors who suddenly start bending it like Beckham. However, based on some studies, there's still a good chance that at least up to the early postmenopausal years, a woman can lower her subsequent risk of breast cancer, not to mention her subsequent risk of colon cancer, by becoming more active.

But there's also this key point. Even if, despite all your best exercising efforts, you develop some malignancy, researchers claim that regular exercise will help you deal better with your disease, especially in managing the many troublesome side effects of the various therapies you may endure.

DIABETES

One of the most important positive effects of exercise is to maintain normal insulin and blood sugar levels, thus lowering the risk of diabetes and reducing the chance of complications in someone who already has diabetes. Finnish researchers estimate that combining an appropriate diet with exercise could prevent 60 percent of all cases of Type 2 diabetes, the most common form of this chronic disease and potential killer. Several studies have concluded that in sedentary adults it may be possible to cut the risk of developing prediabetes with exercise alone, perhaps even if the exercisers don't lose much weight. In the real world, the Nurses' Health Study found that for every two hours of TV watched daily, the risk of diabetes goes up 14 percent. Conversely, watching less than 10 hours of TV a week and going for a brisk half-hour walk every day lowers the risk of diabetes by 43 percent.

It doesn't take much exercise to get this benefit. A single bout of exercise has been shown to lower insulin levels, and hence better glucose levels, an effect that lasts for several hours. Studies have also shown that regular exercise helps maintain better insulin and glucose levels for at least a month after the exercise is discontinued.

But it really shouldn't be surprising that exercise is so effective at combating diabetes. After all, humans were programmed early in evolution to gear up for sudden bursts of energy-sapping activity that might go on for several days at a time. Unlike modern-day workers, who are ready to march home feeling "bushed" after seven hours on the job, many after two hours, our ancestors realized that tracking and killing a mastodon usually didn't happen over a five-hour shift with two 20-minute breaks for coffee and several visits to the washroom to read the morning tabloid. Our forefathers and foremothers simply had to keep going till the killing was done, after which they would gorge and not move for days on end while the plenty lasted—other than to take care of biological business, of course (the closest modern-day model I can think of is adult kids who've moved back home). Those bouts of prolonged labor, however, were bracketed by long bouts of semistarvation (no mastodon, no mastication).

Hence, it makes sense that our genes demand that we do a lot of moving and protect us against times of famine by building up our stores of fat. But now that it's continual feast and hardly any movement for most of us most of the time, our high-energy-related biology goes haywire as a result of our prolonged periods of inactivity and continuous satiety.

These effects can be significantly ameliorated, however, by doing more exercise. In a study from the University of Pittsburgh, 52 overweight adult diabetics who walked for 45 minutes five to six days a week (and received counseling from a registered dietician) lost nearly 10 percent of their body weight, which in turn produced steep falls in their glucose levels, allowing most of those who had been on diabetes medication to discontinue their use of those drugs. That is, enough exercise can allow many diabetics to come off their medications altogether. Another American study showed that exercising three to four times a week significantly lowered the risk status of pre-diabetics.

BRAIN FUNCTIONS

This one may be my trump card. So OK, many of you are willing to risk dying of a heart attack or a stroke because, after all, those are such fast and painless ways to go, right? And many of you are also willing to take your chances with diseases such as breast cancer and colon cancer (after all, man, they're bound to come up with much more effective treatments pretty soon, aren't they?). And I can even accept that many of you are willing to limp along with diabetes (after all, they're coming up with such improved techniques for delivering insulin, aren't they?).

But you know, even my good and gentle and naïve nature can't accept that many of you are willing to have your brains generally deteriorate. So, if you're not enthusiastic about your brain slowly becoming the consistency of a ripe avocado, then, you guessed it, you need to do more exercise. Exercise, you see, offers your brain substantial benefits both in the short term and in the long term.

Short-term benefits
Researchers studied the brains of a group of college students (only students who had actual working brains, of course, so it must have taken the testers a long time to come up with enough study subjects) to find out what effect exercise might have on "thinking ability" in the form of computer tests of varying difficulty. Brain-wave patterns showed that during the most difficult computer tests, exercise not only increased the speed with which these students' brains were able to make decisions about what to answer but also increased the accuracy of their responses. That is, after they exercised, these students not only made decisions slightly faster but also tended to make a larger number of correct decisions. In a similar study, individuals who took up jogging showed consistently improved scores on tests measuring intellectual capacity.

So that's the short-term benefit of being more active—your brain works faster and it works better. "But, wait just a second," some of you will no doubt say. "That's all very well for students who may require fast brains for typical student needs like playing video games and remembering the permutations among all the characters in soap operas. But what about those of us who are, say, street cleaners or lawyers? We don't really need speedy or accurate brains to get along in our worlds, so we're quite happy to do less exercise and maintain our slower, less accurate brains."

Long-term benefits

So let me turn now to the long-term benefits of exercise on that most vital of organs, and we start, of course, with dementia, especially Alzheimer's disease.

Alzheimer's disease is baby boomers' biggest bugaboo. In fact, most people are more afraid of Alzheimer's than they are of death, and to prevent it, most young and midlife adults claim they would do just about anything.

"Anything?"

"Anything."

"Would you take a pill?"

"Anything."

"Do a mental drill?"

"Anything."

"Would you climb a hill?"

"What were the other choices again?"

Yes, you can maintain normal brain function as you age, and exercise helps you do that. A very interesting study found that rats that became addicted to exercise (you can get a rat addicted to anything as long as you feed him enough—which makes rats very similar to teenagers) ended up with healthier brains; rats that ran had better memories and learned new tasks more quickly than those that just sat around and chewed pellets. Another study found that older mice that exercised actually grew new brain cells, while sedentary mice steadily and lazily lost theirs.

Happily, it's not just in rodents that there is a link between more activity and better brain function. We have lots of similar evidence in humans, as well. A study done in Canada found that regular exercisers had a 50 percent lower risk of Alzheimer's and a 40 percent lower risk of all other forms of dementia than those who did not exercise regularly. The harder these exercisers worked, the lower their overall risk of dementia. Another study found that healthy, elderly Swedes lowered their risk of eventual dementia by either leading "active lives"—which, in this study, included participating in activities such as gardening or reading or playing cards (only in Sweden would canasta enthusiasts be considered to be leading active lives)—or by getting regular daily exercise, such as walking and swimming. Older Swedes who got regular physical activity developed dementia at about half the rate over the subsequent six years as did your more typical sedentary senior Swedes.

I must admit, though, that there is another way to interpret the preceding findings, and that is that people who are less prone to dementia in the first place are also more likely to exercise, even at younger ages. Although this interpretation is possible, it is much more probable, I believe, that your brain, like every other organ, is kept younger when you do more physical activity. At the very minimum, we know that exercise:

- Leads to better blood flow to every organ, including the brain, and the more blood an organ receives, the more nourishment it gets and the longer it can maintain its optimum work capacity.
- Lowers blood pressure.
- Leads to more flexible arteries (see above), including cerebral arteries, which also helps the brain.
- Produces higher HDL levels (ditto); low HDL levels have been strongly implicated in the development of dementia.
- Reduces inflammation (which has been associated with dementia).
- Is a sociable activity (lots of data indicate that a rich social life helps protect brain function as we age).

Other brain functions

Finally, if dementia doesn't really worry you (and if it doesn't, may I humbly suggest that might be the first sign of brain deterioration), then you should know that other brain functions are also improved by exercise. According to an American study, seniors who keep active are more "flexible thinkers" than sedentary seniors; active seniors are less easily distracted and can focus better—very useful abilities to maintain, the authors point out, for activities such as driving and shopping for groceries, not to mention the most important one of all, the ability to deal with children who are trying to get you to sign over the family home before you're ready to leave. Even better, seniors who are active, another American study found, are also quicker to respond to situations that need immediate attention, such as the cocoa overheating on the stove.

According to another study, sedentary men and women who were encouraged to get up and start walking showed marked improvement on tests that measured those brain functions known as executive functions, such as planning abilities ("I will watch TV evangelists all day today"), making and remembering choices ("I will have Ovaltine instead of regular cocoa"), and establishing schedules.

And finally, there's this important point: according to the folks who did that last study, the older you are, the more your brain has to gain from doing more exercise.

ERECTILE DYSFUNCTION

Yo, men: this one's for you (well, maybe not for you only, but you know what I mean). Exercise is the best tool to ensure proper working of your tool. The more active a man is, the less he will need to pay attention to those annoying "erection aid" ads that come as spam on his e-mail, thus allowing him to spend more time perusing those penis-enlargement ads instead. Does anyone really read those things? And if you do, take it from me—they never ship you the stuff.

Anyway, according to one study of 600 middle-aged and elderly gents, men who were active were much less likely to develop erectile dysfunction (ED) than were their sit-around bros—even, surprisingly, if the former didn't start to exercise until middle age, a time of life when ED is no longer just a tiny blip on the horizon but rather a too-frequent soft elephant in the bedroom.

And all it took for the men in this study to lower their risk of ED was to expend about 200 calories a day, or what you get from a brisk 3.2 kilometer (2-mile) walk. As you'd expect, however, the more exercise a man does, the lower his risk of erectile difficulties.

A major part of the reason exercise is so beneficial in preventing ED is its blood-vessel-softening effect. Contrary to what you might believe, it's actually the softer, more flexible blood vessels that permit enough blood to gather—and more important, to linger—in the area where you want blood to gather and linger when you're getting pumped and primed for passion. Ergo, run and you will postpone the day that you start humming, "Good morning, good morning, we talked the whole night through..." Talked? Some men need pills for that? Clearly, they're not Jewish.

MOOD AND STRESS LEVELS

Doing exercise is well known to reduce stress levels (see chapter 9). In fact, I believe exercise may be the best stress reliever on the market.

But exercise is also crucial in maintaining a healthy mood or raising your mood when it's low. I'm convinced that there is no better way to improve a bummed-out mood and to raise your energy level than by doing a bit of exercise that at the very least leaves you feeling overbearingly self-righteous and eager to tell your spouse how many reps and rips you just did.

And again, it doesn't take much effort to become more effervescent. In a study that involved a bunch of female college students, who were no doubt selected as subjects because they're about as moody a group as you can find, students who put in at least 10 minutes of moderate exercise just one to three times a week claimed they experienced improved mood and more energy as a result. In another study, from Stanford University, elderly women caregivers who managed to stay with a program of moderate increased activity for one year were "significantly less depressed and stressed" as a result of their new regime. Indeed, regular exercise may be most important as a mood-elevator (the Otis of the psyche) in seniors.

In a study that looked at 1,000 people with an average age of 75, the more exercise these seniors participated in, the better their moods and the better they felt about life in general. Another study found that seniors who were most fit were also the least tired, the least depressed, the least tense, and the least angry. In fact, seniors who had been previously sedentary but who were encouraged to start walking daily responded that they had more "pleasurable feelings" after just a week of walking for 15 minutes once a day.

Exercise also helps reduce anxiety. Researchers from California State University in Chico found that chronic worriers tend to worry less if they work out—as long, I guess, as they don't start to worry about how much exercise they're doing. And exercise has been shown to improve that nebulous concept of "self-esteem," especially in young people, and exercise certainly boosts self-confidence.

Although exercise can help nearly everyone feel better, it may be especially helpful to those who are clinically depressed. Some studies have shown that exercise can be even more effective in fighting depression than antidepressant drugs are. In one small study, people with "severe depression," including some for whom drug therapy had failed completely, were convinced to exercise daily on a treadmill. After as little as 10 days, over half of them reported being "substantially less" depressed, and some others reported being "slightly less" depressed.

◆ ———————————————————————————————— ◆

SOCIAL BENEFITS OF EXERCISE

One of the main benefits of exercise for me is that it makes me more sociable, since going to my workouts gets me out of my home office regularly and into a setting where I meet people and I have to talk to them (while secretly sizing them up to see if I've progressed more than they have). And I am certainly not an isolated case. Exercise should be—and often is—a social activity, one of the most relaxing activities you can do with friends, and as you will read in chapter 9, one of the keys to successful aging is a strong social network.

◆ ———————————————————————————————— ◆

WEIGHT AND BODY SHAPE

Exercise is the best way to lose weight and keep it off. For one thing, exercise burns calories. For another, the more you work out, the more muscle tissue you develop, and even though muscle weighs more than fat, muscle burns calories more efficiently than fat does. Even if you lose weight through dieting, the best way to keep it off as your metabolism adjusts and you start to regain some of what you lost is to do more exercise. Equally important, exercise helps you redistribute your weight—away from "bad" areas, such as the abdomen and (especially good news for men) the chest.

And I am a great advertisement for what I just told you. Until recently, I had always been afraid to bare any parts of my body in public for two main reasons. One, I had—and there really is no better way to phrase this—steadily enlarging "boobs" ("Yes, my dear Watson, men are not supposed to have boobs"). Two, there was my general body shape, a shape my wife once described as remarkably similar to that of a challah, though I preferred to think of myself as a sophisticated French loaf or rye bread (with boobs, of course)—pretty thick from top to bottom, but especially thick around the middle. But with my new workout and weights regime, I now look much more like a baguette, and if not quite a boobless baguette, then at least one with only small onion-bun mammary protrusions. The happy consequence is that I now whip my shirt off in public at the drop of a hat. In fact, I feel so good about myself (I am also a living testament to the benefits of how exercise builds self-esteem) that I often don't even wait for the hat to drop.

As many of you will undoubtedly testify, though, it isn't always easy to lose weight with exercise. Probably because of their genes, some people can't do it at all, or if they do lose weight, it's usually a depressingly pitiful few pounds that are often, alas, too few for anyone of the preferred sex to notice.

So if you're one of those rare people who can't lose a gram of weight despite running 80 kilometers (50 miles) a week, you can take solace from the fact that where you store your fat usually does change as a result. That is by itself a major boon because, the less fat you store around your middle, the better your prognosis.

BONES

Studies show that kids as young as eight or 10 who are very active already have stronger bones than do more sedentary youngsters. This benefit is maintained throughout life, because the more total bone mass young people build up by eating right (getting enough calcium and vitamin D) and by doing enough exercise, the more bony cushion they have to draw on when bone mass inevitably starts to deteriorate during their thirties and forties, and as the process accelerates as the decades pile on.

After the age of 30 or so, exercise can slow the loss of bone that accompanies aging, and it can also increase bone density, which is important in lowering the risk of fracture. To help your bones, however, exercise must be vigorous and weight bearing. So jogging, for example, is much better for your bones than is swimming. Actually, anything is better than swimming—except, of course, golf.

By the way, a recent study that got very little notice found a link between osteoporosis and heart disease. To wit, women with early signs of osteoporosis are up to five times as likely to have heart disease. In this study, osteoporosis was a stronger predictor of heart disease than high blood pressure or diabetes. What's the connection? Well, both conditions have many of the same risk factors, but there may also be an as yet undiscovered metabolic link between the two.

The important point, though, is this: if you have early bone-thinning (often called osteopenia), you may have a higher risk of heart disease (and dementia, according to another study), so have your heart and arteries thoroughly evaluated. More important, do something to lower your risks of these conditions.

JOINTS

Contrary to popular belief, normal exercise does not lead to a higher risk of osteoarthritis (OA), or wear-and-tear arthritis. If you have no injury or abnormality to begin with, racquet sports (played properly) do not lead to OA in the shoulder or elbow, skiing and walking do not lead to deterioration in the hip, and regular jogging does not lead to OA of the knee. Even a lifetime of moderate amounts of running does not lead to joint deterioration in the hip, the knee, the ankle, or the toes. If there's pre-existing injury to a joint, however, or some physical abnormality, then exercise can increase the risk of OA in that joint.

People with OA often complain, understandably, that exercise causes a lot of pain in their inflamed joints. That may indeed be true, but paradoxically, these are the people whose joints probably have the most to gain from being more active. A Dutch study concluded that people with OA of the knee "must" exercise if they want better control of their joint pain and inflammation and if they want less deterioration of their knees.

If you get too much pain from running or even walking, however, non-weight-bearing activities like cycling, swimming, and rowing or reduced-impact exercise using elliptical trainers and stairmasters are other options. Also, single-leg strength work such as working on a leg-press machine can help increase tolerance to weight-bearing exercise if you have OA of the knee.

OTHER BENEFITS

Immune system
Several studies have shown that regular exercise is better than eating right to help keep colds and flus at bay, though very vigorous exercise may impair the immune system slightly. As well, a couple of studies have found that flu vaccine may be more effective in seniors who exercise than in those who don't.

Eating
Another great benefit of exercise that I'm always cashing in on is that exercise allows you to eat more. In a study of young Spanish soccer players, men who played regular soccer weighed less, had more muscle mass, and were able to consume 27 percent more calories a day without gaining weight than a sitting-around peer group. Much of this benefit has to do with all the extra muscle you gain from working out regularly. One calculation I've seen is that if you add 2 kilograms (5 pounds) of muscle, you can consume an extra 250 calories a day.

Independence
The more active you are earlier in life, the more independent and mobile you will be as you reach that age when your kids start advising you to give up your driver's license (usually sometime in your fifties). According to one study, an active 70-year-old had about the same mobility as a sedentary 55-year-old.

Other studies have revealed many other wonderful benefits of exercise, including:

- Better sleep (see chapter 8).
- Increased stamina and endurance.
- Lower risk of asthma and better asthma control.
- Lower risk of back pain.
- Better lung function (one study even claims that exercise was able to reverse a more than 20-year history of declining lung function

within 22 weeks of beginning an activity program).
- Less hospitalization in people who suffer from COPD (chronic obstructive pulmonary disease), especially chronic bronchitis.
- An ability to handle "unexpected challenging activities" (presumably things like your mother coming to visit without the requisite six months' notification).

For young women, there is also the benefit of a longer time between periods (and for all you one-digit-IQ Don Cherry fans, this has nothing to do with playing hockey). With exercise, menstrual periods become more regular and there is a longer time between them, though very heavy exercise can often lead to menstrual disturbances, even a complete loss of periods, resulting in thinner bones. This is an especially severe problem for young, overenthusiastic women athletes and has come to be known as part of the female athlete triad: eating disorders, loss of periods, and stress fractures (with subsequent higher risks of infertility and osteoporosis). So here's a warning to young women: as with everything else in life—food, money, even sex—the key is moderation. Take it from this middle-aged dude: a little bit of most things is good for you, a moderate amount is better, but a whole lot can take you to places you may not really want to go. (The sole exceptions are haggis, ludefisk, head cheese, golf, and anything in aspic, all of which are terrible even in small amounts.)

If It's So Good for You, Why Don't More People Do It?
So if exercise is so good for you, why don't more people do more exercise? Most surveys agree that somewhere around 60 percent of the public admits to being mostly or completely sedentary, and when you eliminate all the liars ("You told those people what they wanted to hear, didn't you, Hubert?"), the morons who have no idea what the interviewers are talking about ("Sure, I get exercised a few times a week"), and those who live in a twilight zone ("Hey! Marge, getting out of bed does so count as a workout"), I'm sure the real percentage of sedentary souls is much higher than these surveys reflect.

Indeed, study after study has shown that people fool themselves about how active they are by inflating the hell out of whatever little activity they manage to get up to. One study, for example, showed that a majority of people who estimated that they generally walked the commonly recommended 10,000 steps a day actually managed to walk closer to 4,000 to 5,000 steps a day according to a pedometer that was strapped onto them. ("Yes, Art, but I take really big steps.")

Bottom line: men and women are simply not active enough. According to a recent survey, only 35 percent of adult men claim to be getting the minimum amount of exercise needed to prevent further deterioration (and we all know how men love to exaggerate their accomplishments, especially their physical ones), while only 30 percent of women claim to be getting that dead rock bottom amount of necessary exercise—and more worrying, the number of women who exercise enough drops significantly with age.

Worst of all, our kids are getting more slothful, too. A recent analysis by University of North Carolina (Chapel Hill) researchers of data on American kids between the ages of 12 and 19 from 1980 to 2000 concluded that obesity has risen by 10 percent, though calorie intake has risen by only 1 percent in that same period. The clear culprit for all that fat is inactivity. Physical activity in teenagers dropped by 13 percent over those two decades.

Sadly, the reason that our kids are growing much more rotundular (to use a term my wife loves) lies with the adults who control kids' lives. Kids today are driven to school by their parents instead of being made to walk (in my day, it was uphill both ways, of course, in the snow and through swarms of mosquitoes), kids are involved in far more after-school activities that are primarily sedentary (choir, language lessons, etc.) than was the case in our day (my only after-school activity consisted of being forced to walk my brother home from school), and perhaps most important, kids are no longer allowed to play in unsupervised settings (I still remember the tackle football games we played on the only playing surface near our house, which also happened to be paved—toughens you up, though).

So kids today have relatively inactive childhoods, but at least one can forgive them because kids don't know better. Adults, however, presumably have much more control over their lives than kids do, and adults should know better, so why are most adults such sluggards? One clear reason is that we don't want to put out the effort. True, there are a few notable exceptions, endorphin-crazed individuals who actually enjoy the "work" part of a workout, but the majority of people are like my son, who much prefers the "out" part.

Even worse, most of us are also supremely lazy in our daily lives. For one of my several jobs (I have several jobs, but my wife still tells everyone, "Arthur? Oh, he's retired"; I can't help it if the trend is to work at home, near the fridge), I have to occasionally show up in a large downtown building in Vancouver, and let me tell you that it is an extremely rare sight to see anyone walk the one flight of stairs from the parking lot to the lobby. The only people who do walk look fit; the overweight often wait a minute or two for the extremely slow elevator rather than take the stairs. They also prefer to wait for a parking spot as close to the elevator as they can find rather than walk 45 meters (50 yards) from their car.

But most people would never offer up their sloth as an explanation for their lack of activity and backside backsliding, and claim they would be more active if only:

- They had more time.
- Working out were more fun.
- They weren't so old (this often comes from people in their twenties or thirties).
- They didn't have a pre-existing condition that prevents them from doing any exercise ("My rabbi doesn't think I should run, Art").
- Exercise were not so fraught with peril and danger and not so potentially injurious.
- They didn't have to do "so much" to regain the fitness level they had when they were younger ("You can't believe how fit I once was, Art").

So let's tackle some of those excuses, oops, I mean, "reasons."

Lack of time. It just doesn't take that much time to get enough exercise to lower your risk of disease. I mean, we're only talking 30 minutes four times a week, folks, or to use my maths again, two hours out of a total of 168 during a week. So even if you add in preparation time (after all, it takes at least 39 seconds to tie your shoelaces, and about a minute more to change your undies and put on running shorts—if you change your undies, that is), that's still less than three hours a week.

Now, I don't know how most of you live, but I do know that you can certainly find three hours a week to take from something else and donate to your health if you want to. Get up 30 minutes earlier, for example, or spend 30 minutes less a night on *The Sopranos* or *Survivor: Trapped in Toledo* or any of those other mindless but sedentary activities you do manage to find time for. After all, the average North American spends an astonishing equivalent of 57 days a year watching TV—and that's only an average, meaning that some North Americans watch way more TV than that. And this figure doesn't include all those hours so many of us waste in front of computers and playing video games.

The time is there; you just have to apportion it properly by making exercise a priority.

To make it even more convenient, the mavens of movement now say that it's even OK to do workouts in 10-minute sessions. So if you truly can't find a half-hour to spare on a Sunday, for example, you can get away with three 10-minute sessions at any time during that day of rest—say, one right before your brunch, one a couple of hours after you eat (after all, we don't want you straining your full tummy with all that lox and cream cheese in it), and then maybe one 10-minuter while the TV is warming up later in the afternoon.

The exercise experts are also willing to count just about any activity as contributing to overall fitness levels. Taking this trend to what I consider an extreme, a study found that most domestic activities such as lawn-mowing and even window-cleaning, for heaven's sake, could be counted as moderate bursts of activity for fitness purposes, though for some reason, flower-arranging and vacuuming did not count (so why do they call it "power-vacuuming?" I ask).

Know one great trick for finding the time, by the way? Prepay for it. You'd be amazed at how often I'm certain I can't get out of bed, let alone get to my workout class at the ungodly hour of 8 AM, until I realize (usually because my wife is yelling at me) that I've paid good money for this, and I'm going to lose that money if I don't get there. It's amazing how the time and energy suddenly materialize.

Exercise is not fun. That depends entirely on how you define "fun." True, exercise is never as much fun as say, watching Cameron Diaz do something, but it can still be pleasurable, especially when you begin to see some progress, and you will see progress—less weight, better aerobic capacity, more strength—if you just stick with it.

Exercise is also invariably more fun if you do it with someone else, even if that someone is a low-life fascist trainer who revels in watching you slowly dehydrate and melt in front of him. So run with a roomie, bend with a buddy, stretch with a sister, flex with a friend, or walk with a wife or husband. Exercising with a friend or trainer is also likely to get you to stick to your schedule more than you might on your own.

Too old to exercise. If you're not too old to contemplate having sex (you don't actually have to do it—"Whew!"—you just have to think about doing it), then you're not too old to start exercising. Doctors don't agree about much, but there's complete consensus on at least one point: there are benefits to starting an exercise program at any age. Indeed, the older you are, the more you probably have to gain from exercise.

Too unhealthy to exercise. Very few health conditions should prevent you from doing some type of exercise. Most health problems are actually ameliorated by exercise, and if not ameliorated, then at the very least made more tolerable. Studies have shown that people suffering from chronic fatigue syndrome, for example, do better if they start to be more active, that people with irritable bowel syndrome manage better if they exercise, that people with all types of arthritis tend to complain of less pain if they become more active, and even that soldiers suffering from Gulf War syndrome complain of less fatigue and have better mental health and better physical functioning if they do enough exercise. True, some conditions (an amputation of a limb, for example) limit the kinds of exercise you can choose. But for nearly everyone, there are activites that can be pursued.

Too dangerous. For those who argue that they won't exercise because they fear dying during their activity, well, yes, sudden intense activity such as shoveling snow or mowing the lawn or moving the couch can kill you. There are, however, two ways to deal with that threat to life: (1) hire someone else to do the work for you, or, and this is a much better choice, (2) get fit. You see, the more fit you become, the lower your risk that a sudden intense burst of activity will do you in. Number two is also a better choice for most of us because as long as there are spouses there will always be couches to move and lawns to mow and boxes to tote and you can't always find someone to do those jobs for you (at least, that's how I convinced my wife to get more fit). So if you don't become fit, the threat of sudden death from exertion will forever be hanging over your head. It's been estimated that a fit man of 50 has about a 1 in 1.5 million chance of dying from sudden exertion, but those odds are a hundred times higher for a male who is mostly sedentary.

Takes too long to reach an acceptable fitness level. To this one I have only two things to say. First, Dallas. Yes, Dallas. Big *D*, little *a*, double *l-a-s*. Remember the Dallas Bed Rest and Training Study? Well, if you don't, it just proves my point that you need to be more active to maintain or retrain your brain. Anyway, in that study, out-of-shape 50-year-old Texans were able to regain nearly the same excellent fitness level they had at the age of 20 with only six months of fitness training. So it doesn't take long to become fit.

Second, you don't have to aim for a high level of fitness to get lots of benefit out of exercising because, as the exercise experts never tire of reminding us, the amount of exercise needed for health benefits is considerably less than the amount of exercise needed to become physically fit, which is why the experts all agree: the biggest gains from exercise accrue to those who just start to do any exercise at all.

CHAPTER

2

Getting Started

The Road to Well Is Paved
with Good Exertions

I recently turned 60. Practically a third of my life
is nearly over.
WOODY ALLEN, "Sayings of the Week," *The Observer*

S O, WE'VE ARRIVED at the point in this book, I figure, where some of you are just chomping at the bit to get more active, though lots of others, alas, are simply chomping on bacon bits. For those who need more prodding, here's an old joke that will maybe spur you to become more active, because it might just save your lives.

Two guys are walking in the woods when they come face-to-face with an angry bear. One guy starts shaking and crying that there's no way out, but the other guy calmly doffs his backpack and takes out his runners, which he starts to put on.

"Are you crazy?" says guy number one. "You can't outrun a bear."

"I know," says guy number two. "But I can outrun you."

Hey, you never know, but before charging off to a workout class, hold your horses just a bit longer, pardner, because there are still a couple of key issues to deal with.

First, how much exercise do you need to do to be healthy? Depends on whom you believe.

You see, there are two schools of thought. The Exercise Lite School believes that a minimal to moderate amount of exercise gives you nearly as much protection as a whole lot of exercise does. The Bop Till You Drop School believes that although a moderate amount of exercise confers modest health benefits, the greatest benefits by far accrue to those who participate in the most vigorous types of activity.

The Exercise Lite people can cite several studies supporting their beliefs, showing, for example, that high-intensity exercise confers only a slightly lower risk of premature death than moderate-intensity exercise, that the greatest gains in longevity occur in men who go from no fitness to some fitness, or that walking slowly for an hour a day is nearly as good as running in reducing the risk of heart disease. But the Bop Till You Droppers, of whom I am one, can point to a study of over 44,000 male physicians that found that those men who exercised the hardest had the lowest risk of heart disease, and that there was no reduced risk of heart disease for men who participated in only light activity such as ambling no matter how much time they spent doing it. Or we can point to that Welsh study cited earlier that found no reduction in mortality rate from light exercise such as walking but a substantial benefit from heavy exercise such as running.

So the findings conflict a lot, as do their proponents. What should you do then? Whatever you like. Do something, anything, and you'll get some benefits. Do more, and it's likely you'll get more benefits. Do a lot, and perhaps you will get the most benefits. But start with something.

There is one special case, though, that I have to note before continuing. Sadly, there indeed seem to be some people who don't seem to get fit no matter how hard they work at it, people who are neither liars nor closet sluggards but simply folks who, based on some kind of genetic abnormality, can work out a hell of a lot with very little gain. If that's you, just skip to the next section. But before you all rush off to include yourselves in that group, know that I just don't believe you, nor will most people.

How Long, O Lord, How Long Before I See Results?

The good news is that it doesn't take that long at all to get some health benefits from exercise. I've already told you a couple of times about those Good Old Boys in Dallas who took only about six months to regain an excellent fitness level. Dallas is not unique. In another study, 30 minutes of brisk walking a day for five to six times a week lowered the participants' risk of heart attack by 25 percent within six months of beginning the program.

But hey, if six months sounds as if it's still too long, then take heart in this: one study of 11 obese men found that three weeks after they'd started on a moderate exercise regime of walking on a treadmill, they experienced noticeable improvements in several markers of disease, even though the men had not lost any weight. (Yes, they were supposed to be on a diet, but the food was offered buffet style, and since these are guys and the food was unlimited and the meals were unsupervised... well, you know why they didn't lose weight.) But the thing is that within three weeks, these fat guys were already benefiting from just doing a bit more.

A word of warning, though: like the Italian army, this effect also kicks into reverse quickly, so if, say, you're a regular midlife exerciser who decides to abandon his exercise regime, within six months of taking up your new prone position on the couch, you will raise your risk of having a heart attack by 25 percent.

I Just Can't, I Really, Really Can't

For those of you who don't have the time or simply can't set up an exercise schedule, the fitness experts have all sorts of suggestions as to how to add even a bit more activity to your daily routine:

- At work, instead of e-mailing your colleagues, deliver your message in person.
- Instead of meeting a business crony for lunch, take him or her for a walk around the building.
- How about taking a brisk, 10-minute walk before breakfast or after dinner?

- Park the car as far away as you can when visiting a mall to do your shopping so that you can schlep the groceries farther (that's both aerobics and resistance training, you see).
- Walk to work or to the store instead of taking the car.
- Use the stairs rather than the elevators—a tactic that surely would be beneficial to my radio coworkers, since our offices are located on the 21st floor of our building. I always use the stairs for anything to a maximum of three flights up and six flights down, and for the Type A's out there, let me tell you that it's invariably quicker to walk it.
- Some experts even suggest doing calisthenics while you're talking on the phone or watching TV. Hey, don't blame me, folks, I just report these suggestions. I'm with you, though, and I too wonder if any of the bozo experts who come up with this kind of stuff really believe that anyone who's watching *Larry King Live* is actually going to start doing crunches in the middle of the program.

The bottom line is just to move more and not to use all the technological tools that are available to limit your physical effort. In short, I'll again cite the brilliant words of the late fitness guru Dr. George Sheehan, who once said something like this: "All you need to be fit is to live in a two-story house and have a very poor memory." Which also partially explains, by the way, why I am becoming so much more fit as I get older.

Enough Already: How Do I Start?

If you're anywhere near middle age or older, if you have a health condition, or if you've been a lifelong recalcitrant reclining russet, *see your doctor before embarking on a new exercise program* to get a pre-exercise evaluation from her about your present state of health and what, if any, limitations it might impose on you. Your doctor, if she's smart and doesn't want a lawsuit from your eventual inheritors, will evaluate the state of your arteries and heart and the level of your blood pressure, then do appropriate tests (a stress ECG is a very good idea if you've never engaged in sports before or if you have any risk factors for sudden death), especially if you're middle-aged or beyond. Depending on the results, she will then advise you about how vigorous an exercise regime you should attempt and how quickly you can adjust your output.

Once you've received your exercise clearance, you then have to:

- *Determine what it is you want from an exercise regime.* If you want to lose weight, you might choose different exercises from what you would select to merely lessen your long-term risk of heart disease.
- *Make a long-term plan.* And I don't just mean make a schedule, though that's important. The trouble with schedules, however, is that they break down very easily, and a bad PMS day, or a bad hair day, or a bad conversation with your mother can often lead to a change in your schedule for that day. A plan, however, makes you think long-term about where you want to get and what you need to do to get there.
- *Be patient and be reasonable about your expectations.* Or to quote my son, "Don't be so damn anal." Unfortunately, this is where far too many people screw up: they set unachievable goals and unrealistic schedules, and they quit when they can't measure up to their bloated expectations. That's why, of course, over half the people who start an exercise program stop within a few weeks. So listen up, folks. Not only is there lots of pleasure in just doing the exercise, but hey, it took you 40 or 50 years to become the blimp you see every morning in the bathroom mirror, so it's just common sense that it's going to take a while to make you become more svelte. And skipping a day or two is not going to undermine your long-term goals.
- *Get a buddy to join you in your new routine, preferably someone who is starting out, too.* Most people look to their spouses first, but speaking from personal experience, I'm not sure that's such a great idea. It's not likely, for example, that you and your spouse will be able to accommodate the same exercise schedule—who's doing the dishes when you're both out running, eh? Besides, what if you and your spouse progress at different rates? I don't know about your relationship, but mine would certainly not be able to stand the stress if I ever ran any distance faster than my wife could. Luckily, I can't.
- *Join a fitness club if you can't find a buddy.* Again, if you pay money for something, you're more likely to stick with it.
- *Start at a level that isn't uncomfortable—or more accurately, not too uncomfortable—and build slowly.* In other words, and as my wife often admonishes me, start low and go slow. But as soon as it feels

easy, take things up a notch. Although exercise experts no longer adhere to the principle of "no pain, no gain," you can bet the farm that if you're not working up a sweat, you're not going to make much progress, and if your progress is very slow, I can also bet that you won't stick with your regime for very long.

- *Set aside adequate time to engage in your chosen activity on a frequent and regular basis.* Sure, you get the same total time of exercise from running two hours every Saturday as you do from running a half-hour every Monday, Wednesday, Friday, and Sunday, but you know, you will get a whole lot more benefit from the latter schedule, with much less risk of injury. You really don't want to be a weekend warrior, one of those many people, usually of the guy persuasion, who does very little during the week except attend meetings and sip martinis, then spends the weekend trying to make up for that lack of activity. Not only does that kind of pattern lead to a much higher risk of injury, it also—horrors!—leads to a higher risk of dying suddenly during the intense physical activity.

So Many Choices, So Little Time

So what should you choose? This is a very crucial matter because you are only going to succeed in an exercise program if you like what you are doing. It's no good picking swimming, for example, if, like me, you're not at all into water sports.

So pick something you like. This seems like common sense, but you'd be amazed at how many people get involved in some activity—snowshoeing, for example, or hang-gliding—just because they've heard it's the "best" one to do or because they have a friend who's already doing it. And for heaven's sake, no matter what you do, *don't choose golf.* Golf is not a sport, it's certainly not exercise, and just as certainly it doesn't do anything to extend your life expectancy. As a Jewish friend says, "Golf is only attractive to men who like to brag about their long putts." And I'm not just golf-bashing again. In a study that followed male medical students from young adulthood through middle age, the researchers found that although sports such as tennis correlated with much better rates of heart disease, golf had absolutely no beneficial effect (probably because golfer-doctors drive golf carts rather than walk the course). In contrast, walking, jogging, hiking, cycling, swimming, and cross-country skiing are all good choices.

Invest in Good Equipment

Another piece of advice from someone who's been there and done that: buy some equipment to use at home. Often, it will get you working when nothing else will. That treadmill in my workout room, for example, always awakens a guilty feeling when I pass by it and see it sitting lonely and unused, so I often fire it up just to ease those guilt pangs. The other reason I believe so strongly in treadmills is that they're exactly like wives: you simply cannot lie to a treadmill. Although it's easy to cheat on how hard you've pushed yourself on a run along the beach—something I've frequently done—it's impossible to cheat on a treadmill, which humorlessly monitors your distance, your time, and your effort. In one study, women who used a treadmill as part of their exercise regime lost twice as much weight as women who were allowed to keep track of their exercise on their own.

And make bloody sure you have the right equipment for the activity you've chosen. If you're determined to jog or run, don't scrimp on your runners, though you certainly don't need a $300 pair of brand-name runners, either. But running or walking in good shoes that you replace frequently (not once every two years, as my son does, and then only because the soles have come completely off) is important. A good rule is to replace your runners every 400 kilometers (250 miles) or so—if you manage to run that far, of course.

Socks are also important. In fact, I'm so partial to my feet that although it kills me, I actually pay $14 for special two-layer running socks. And what applies to runners and socks applies even more to other equipment: make sure it's the right equipment and the best you can afford for what you want to achieve.

My most valuable piece of exercise equipment, by the way, may very well be my trainer, even though he costs a ton (like a good hooker, he only rents by the hour, and he doesn't want anything to do with you after he's given you what you paid him to do), and even though he's about as funny as my malamute (I take that back: Big Louie is definitely funnier). My trainer's value lies elsewhere, however. He not only keeps me on track but also shows me the right way to do everything. There definitely is a right way to lift a weight, for example, and a wrong way to lift a weight, and given my abilities, my temperament, and my genetic makeup, I invariably pick the wrong way if left to do it on my own. My trainer, however, continually corrects my posture and makes sure I actually use my abs during crunches, and on and on.

So if you can afford it, folks, invest in some face time with a personal trainer. And remember: whatever you pay him, in the end, he'll cost you less than a funeral (though strictly speaking, I suppose, you don't really pay for your own funeral).

Also, be careful around equipment. Honestly, I once witnessed someone drop a multipound weight on his toes, and hey, it still hurts when it rains. Just kidding, because for once, it wasn't me but rather someone who ordinarily isn't clumsy. He was distracted for a moment, and the next thing he knew he was the owner of a fractured toe. And for God's sake, be especially careful with kids who are allowed anywhere near exercise equipment. Talk to anyone who works in an emergency department and you will hear horror stories of kids who caught their hands in treadmills or stationary bikes or who fell off benches onto their heads. So, if you have exercise equipment at home, that room should be out-of-bounds for kids and clumsy klutzes. That's the rule my wife has for our house, by the way, and it works, too—though I wish she would let me in there once in a while.

One sport in which proper equipment may be especially important is biking. According to some rather scary reports, men who bike lots tend to suffer from pelvic pain, impotence, sexual dysfunction, sperm abnormalities, and infertility (I hope some of you guys didn't fall off your stationary bikes while you were reading this). There is little proof yet that those "anatomically friendly" special seats that are supposed to take the pressure off the nether parts actually lower the risk of those pee-pee problems, but they certainly can't hurt. According to at least one expert, women cyclists also suffer from pelvic pain and sexual dysfunction, as well as pain with intercourse, as a result of biking, so women may also benefit from "anatomically friendly" bike seats. Bottom line: male or female, if you do lots of biking, buy a good bike (perhaps even with shocks), get set up properly on the bike (many bike stores offer this service), buy yourself a good seat and a good helmet, and most important, have your kids sooner rather than later.

Finally, if you're not into spending any money on equipment, I can attest that one of the best pieces of "exercise equipment" in our house is Big Louie, the world's dumbest malamute, who, rain or snow or sleet or whatever, still needs his two walks a day. Let me tell you, when you have Big Louie on a leash, you get a workout.

No One Said It Was Going to Be Quick

No one but you can really gauge how quickly you can and should increase your distance, pace, stroke capacity, etc., but here are some tips:

- *Use your common sense to decide how hard to push yourself.* If you try to do too much too fast, you're undoubtedly going to develop an overuse syndrome (pain and inflammation from the overuse of a muscle group, or even a stress fracture), and then all your lovely plans will be back to square one. Exercise experts commonly advise that you not increase your intensity more than 10 percent every week and that you even reduce your intensity every fourth or fifth week before resuming your regular pace.
- *Vary your workouts.* Several studies have shown that just as with sex, people who vary their exercise regime are more likely to stick with it than those who are always into the same old same old.
- *If you're trying to lose weight, it may benefit you to vary the intensity of each workout, too.* In at least one study, reported in the journal *Medicine and Science in Sports and Exercise,* men who varied their pace when running lost more weight and more fat after 10 weeks than did those men who kept to one steady pace.
- *Drink water.* All the experts agree: water can't harm you and it might actually do you some good. Sticking with my commitment to be completely honest, however, I confess that I drink only occasionally during a workout (except when I want a break from my trainer) and never on a run (I run 8 or 9 kilometers, 5 or 6 miles), and I doubt that it makes any difference to either my times or my enjoyment. So sure, you need some water, and I would never dissuade you from drinking as much as you feel you need, but if you're not thirsty,

seems to me you don't really need to worry about it. When you work out in hot weather, however, especially if you are getting on in years, do make sure to drink lots of water so that you don't dehydrate. This is particularly important to everyone who runs in warm, humid conditions, since heat stroke can be fatal.

- *Stretch if you feel like it.* Everyone says that you must stretch before exercising and warm up properly. I agree that you should warm up slowly and ease into your workout by gradually increasing the intensity of your effort. I don't agree, however, with those who say that you must stretch as part of your warm-up. The only studies I've seen that tried to measure the effects of stretching found inconsistent results concerning the risk of muscle pull or the amount of pain the athlete had after the exercise (see below). That said, I love stretching after a run or workout. It just feels so good.
- *Once you decide to do the work, don't let things get in your way.* It's easy to allow normal daily distractions to interfere with your exercise plans, and you generally should not allow that to happen. Make exercise a priority, not an easily postponable dalliance.
- *Have patience.* If you start to exercise in order to lose weight, and you don't see quick results, don't lose heart, because your heart is getting some benefit, anyway. Just keep reminding yourself that most experts concur that fat, fit people still do far better health-wise than people who are thin and not fit.
- *Finally, keep with it.* You will improve. And you can learn to like exercise; you just have to stick with it long enough for those endorphins to kick in. For me, it took over 20 years. I've been running since my early thirties (it's on DVD—*Run, Artie, Run*), but I only learned to really like it when I reached my early fifties. Now, I love running, and not just because, as my wife says, I can be so smug and self-righteous about it. It really has become fun.

Take Up Irresistible Resistance Training

You're not going to believe what I'm about to tell you, but here it is, anyway: the part of my exercise regime that I enjoy the most is lifting weights. See? I knew you wouldn't believe me, but it's true. I love sweating all over those dumbbells—not just over the trainers, but over the equipment, too.

HOT TIP

The more adventurous might want to imbibe coffee with honey before working out. Several studies have demonstrated that drinking coffee before physical activity can lead to an improvement in performance, and a couple of studies have demonstrated that honey can give your workout a jolt, too. Too much coffee, however, will precipitate wasteful visits to the toilet.

Why do I enjoy it so much? Partly because my biceps have begun to bulge. (Well, that may be an exaggeration, but at the very least, they are burgeoning bubbles.) Not only that, if you have good eyesight and look really, really hard when I flex my arms, you can also see the faint outline of triceps on the backs of my arms.

What's more, I have even developed the very slightest hint of pec definition where my boobs used to be, or to be honest, where my boobs still hang out, though they don't hang out nearly as much as they used to. Weight training has also helped me redistribute fat from around my midsection to, well, I'm not really sure where it's gone (my wife says it's moved to my brain, but I don't think so since my brain doesn't feel any heavier), but a lot of it has disappeared from around my middle, which is quite unlike what's happened to most of you, I'm sure.

You see, by the age of 70, according to one study, unless you do something about it, you will have lost at least 20 percent of the muscle mass you had managed to build up at age 30. The same study found that 70 percent of senior women and 35 percent of senior men can't lift even 4.5 kilograms (10 pounds).

What's worse, muscle cells lost with age are replaced by fat, and your metabolism also slows as you grow older. You can readily see, then, why as you age, you tend to gain weight (usually lots of weight) even if you don't increase how much you eat.

OK, enough bad news, as I regularly tell my mother during our phone calls (Jewish mothers mostly phone when they have bad news, usually something about the underachieving son of a friend of theirs), so let me

tell you that there are, happily, two ways—a good way, and a bad way—
to deal with age-related muscle loss and fat accumulation.

First, the bad way (well, I'm my mother's son, after all). Some "anti-
aging experts" assure us, and many people have grasped at this with un-
seemly haste, that at least some of that age-related muscle loss and fat

WHAT ABOUT HEART RATE?

Most experts want you to monitor your heart rate while you're working out
because that should allow you to gauge how hard you're actually working and
may also keep you from venturing into or lingering in an exercise danger
zone where, in theory, you increase your risk of dying suddenly. But I'm not
sure if that's necessary or even desirable. Heart rate monitors may allow elite
athletes to gauge how hard they're working, but I know of no studies showing
that wearing a heart rate monitor prevents run-of-the-mill athletes like you
and me from suffering a heart attack or dying suddenly during exercise. Besides, I continually register out of the heart rate target zone when working
out, which I attribute to an overactive sympathetic nervous system. (The
easy-to-figure-out-while-you're-exercising formula is 220 minus your age,
multiplied by 60 to 75 percent.) I am sure there are many others like me who
would be prevented from working out as hard as they like if their sessions
were governed solely by the use of a heart rate monitor (after all, most fitness
instructors would be loath—for legal reasons, if nothing else—to permit
their clients to continue working out above the desirable heart rate).

I also believe that wearing a heart rate monitor may give some of you a
false sense of security. There are probably some people out there who might
ignore important warning signs of heart problems, such as chest pain, if
they're wearing a monitor that keeps registering desirable readings. However,
as with everything else in the medical business, the final answer is up to you,
so if you feel more comfortable or safer with a heart rate monitor, then by all
means, get one. (And if you are at higher risk of suffering a heart attack during physical activity, you also ought to discuss the use of a heart rate monitor
with your doctor.) Yes, that is my final answer.

accumulation can be reversed with hormone potions and injections, "anti-aging" prescriptions that cost a fortune and must be continued for, well, for the rest of your life, of course. Depending on which experts you consult, these concoctions include any or all of several hormones, such as human growth hormone, testosterone, and dehydro-epiandrosterone (DHEA, a "cousin" to testosterone and estrogen), as well as other "anti-aging" chemicals.

The problem is that there is little evidence to back these claims.

Take the change in muscle mass that accompanies the use of growth hormone. Yes, one small, very frequently cited study of senior gents showed that growth hormone injections lead to more muscle mass and less fat, but other studies have indicated that new muscle mass from growth hormone doesn't actually lead to any gain in strength. In fact, growth hormone injections can lead to significant problems with tissue swelling (such as carpal tunnel syndrome) as well as a very high rate of insulin resistance.

Further, there is no good evidence that any of these therapies improve quality of life (a recent small study on DHEA, for example, found no benefit in boosting memory) or, more to the point, extend life.

And perhaps most important, there is no proof at all that these anti-aging therapies are safe in the long term. At least one good study found that nearly half the men who received growth hormone injections in a bid to reverse muscle loss developed unhealthy spikes in their blood sugar levels soon after going on this regime—a trend, the researchers worried, that might get even worse the longer the men received those injections. And no one really knows the longer-term effects of such a program (cancer, anyone?). After all, even "normal" doses of hormones can raise the risk of cancer (especially if the hormones are taken for a long time), as women who were urged to take hormone replacement therapy for menopause are now discovering. So what do you think might happen if, over two decades from, say, your fifties or sixties, you were to take regular injections of a hormone that's supposed to make tissue grow? I, for one, don't want anyone to do those experiments on me.

Now, the good news. A much better way to deal with age-related tissue redistribution is with resistance training, which not only replaces fat with muscle (meaning you are not inevitably condemned to looking like a domed stadium from the side). Resistance training does not only

mean weight training. It means pushing or pulling against some form
of resistance, and that can come from weights, from towels, from thera-
bands (those neat rubber bands with handles that look like they'd make
great slingshots) or, most significantly, from your own body weight,
which means that you can exercise many of your major muscle groups
in the comfort of your own home, without using equipment.

RECIPE FOR RESISTANCE EXERCISE

Two terms that you need to learn to do resistance training are *reps* and *sets*.
Reps is short for repetitions, and refers to the number of repetitions of a
particular exercise you do in a row. A set is the total number of reps that you
do without stopping. So if you are doing three sets of 15 reps in a particular
exercise, it means that you do 15, rest for a short period, do 15 more, rest
again, and then do the final 15.

The first exercise I recommend is the push-up. This helps strengthen and
tone the chest (pectorals), the shoulders, and the triceps (the muscles on
the backs of your arms). You can do push-ups either from your toes or from
your knees as long as you keep your body straight. Put your hands on the
floor at the level of your shoulders but just outside of them. Press yourself
straight up (again, either on your knees or on your toes), keeping your body
perfectly straight, as if there were a board running the length of your body
from your chin to your knees (or toes). Don't let your hips drop to the floor
(this is hard on your lower back), and don't push your butt high in the air—
this minimizes the effectiveness of the push-up, changes the focus from
your chest to your front shoulders, and most important, looks silly. Lower
your body back to the floor, but don't rest—keep yourself about 5 to 7 centimeters (2 to 3 inches) off the ground. Congratulations! You just did one
rep! Aim to do two to three sets of 15 to 20 reps.

The next exercise that I recommend for beginners is the squat. Squats
focus on the butt muscles and the muscles in the fronts of your legs (the
quadriceps). This exercise may seem easy to do, but the key is to do it right.
The best way to ensure that you are doing squats correctly is to stand facing
a wall, with your toes 1 inch away from the base, and with your toes and
knees lined up straight ahead. Put your hands on your hips, or keep them

just in front of your shoulders if it helps you to balance. Slowly lower your
butt down as if you were going to take a seat, keeping the weight back on
your heels and not on your toes. Focus your eyes straight ahead as you lower
yourself, keep your shoulders pulled back, and make sure your knees never
go forward over your toes (this is what the wall is there for). You want to try
to get your thighs perpendicular to the floor, and then come back up to full
height. Stick with it, and if the only way you can do it is if you don't go down
far to start, so be it. You will get better with time. Also, try to keep the speed
with which you do squats to a minimum—two to three seconds on the way
down, about two seconds on the way up. Again, aim to do two to three sets
of 15 to 20 reps.

Another good resistance exercise you can do at home is the basic
crunch. To do a crunch, you may want to put down a thin mat (you can find
these in the fitness section of almost any department store) or just use the
carpet. Place your feet flat on the floor, with your toes against the wall. Put
your arms behind your ears, or across your chest, but wherever you put
them, bear in mind that you do not want to pull your head up with your
hands. Keeping your chin off your chest, *slowly* roll your upper body from the
floor until your shoulder blades come up. Then slowly lower yourself down.
It may seem like a very small movement, but that's okay, because it's not
meant to be big.

Try to do two sets of 15 reps every couple of days.

One final instruction: don't hold your breath while you do any resistance
exercise. The easiest way to remember to ensure you don't is to breathe out
when you are exerting yourself (i.e., when you push yourself up in the push-
up), and breathe in while you relax the muscles (when you lower yourself in
the push-up).

There you go! Keep at these exercises for a few weeks, and you'll feel
ready and confident to step up to the next level.

◆ ——————————————————— ◆

In addition to helping you build muscles, resistance training has been
shown to have all sorts of other physical benefits:

• A 13-year study of Canadian men found that an excellent determinant of their longevity was—wait for it—the strength of their

abdominal muscles; the men who could do the most crunches had about half the death rate of the men who could do the fewest.

- Resistance training has been linked to reduced risks of heart attack and diabetes. A huge study of male health professionals found that men who lifted weights for 30 minutes or more per week had a 23 percent reduction in risk of heart attack. Another study found that high-intensity resistance training improved insulin sensitivity, meaning that people doing such training were less likely to develop diabetes (and high blood pressure), and perhaps cancer, too.
- Resistance training has been shown to burn lots of extra calories. According to one study, women who did resistance training had higher metabolism and energy expenditure for two hours after the training was done.
- Even better, the more muscle you have, the more you can eat, since adding 2 kilograms (5 pounds) of muscle allows an average guy (bearing in mind, of course, that the average guy will never put on 2 kilos of muscle) 250 extra calories a day.
- Resistance training can also improve your balance, as I have happily discovered, because the stronger your muscles, the more easily you can maintain your balance. This benefit is especially important in seniors, for preventing falls (a very common source of disability and even death for the elderly).
- It can reduce your risk of osteoporosis and future fractures. In one study, the more weight women lifted over the course of a year, the better the bone density in their hips—a huge benefit to the women, in that hip fractures kill 20 percent of the people who get them.
- Resistance training can improve energy levels.
- In men, it can lower the risk of ED. The more fat a man carries, the higher his risk of ED, so becoming leaner through resistance training and replacing fat with muscle can lead to better performance in a place where every man wants to give the best performance he can. Besides, if you look good, you get more chances to perform.
- But wait, folks, I've saved the best inducement for last. The pièce de résistance is that if you do enough resistance training, you might end up with great legs! It's true. Several women—well, two, and one is very nearsighted and wasn't wearing her glasses at the time—have

come up to me during exercise class to tell me they think I have great legs. And yes, I'm sure it wasn't some sort of sorority stunt.

So those are some physical benefits from resistance training. There are lots of others benefits, too, such as:

- A change in your exercise from time to time as you work out aerobically makes the rest of your exercise regime feel more manageable. I mean, there's just so much running or other aerobic activity anyone can—or ought to—do.
- If you're a Type A personality, one of the beautiful things about resistance training is that you can chart the incremental improvements you make from month to month (OK, from year to year). You have no idea how wonderful it feels when the trainer finally says, "OK, Art, let's go from two pounds to two and a half pounds today." That feeling fades pretty quickly, of course, when you can't lift that new, heavier weight, but hey, you strut until you fail.
- Weight training also makes aerobics easier. That's an important reason why all athletes who compete in aerobic sports also do weight lifting to build muscles, even in muscle groups that seemingly have little importance to their chosen sport.

Don't Wait to Start Weights, But Start Them Right

It may surprise you to learn that few studies have been done about how often one should do weights, how quickly one should increase the amount being lifted, how quickly one should lift a particular set of weights (my trainer is always after me to "slow down, Art, slow down, this is not a race," but hey, the faster you lift them, the faster you get them down, too), whether it's better to do free weights as opposed to machine weights, how many sets to do, how to move between sets, and so on.

One trend in New York these days (now that pashminas are so last year; what is a pashmina, anyway?) is to do—are you ready—eight minutes of weight training once a week. If you do it right, says the eight-minutes-per-week guru, you can stop doing all other forms of exercise, including aerobics, and still get fit. All you have to do over those eight whole minutes is pay a man a lot of money while he watches you slowly lift the absolute maximum weight you can manage. In a city where the average denizen has an attention span of about eight minutes, this latest fast-fitness craze has really taken off.

Like you, I really wish it were that simple to get fit, but until someone does a study that compares eight-minutes-per-week lifters with people who work out for longer, I'll stick with what we know actually works: a steady and slow increase in resistance training.

Rule number one for resistance training is learn to do it properly. Don't just try to lift what you can (unless you live in New York); always remember that as with sex, it's not how rapidly you get there (within reason, of course) but how well you do it that really matters. Technique is all, in other words, which means that you have to get someone who knows what they're doing to teach you how to do it right. And just as important, someone who knows what they're doing should keep watching you, because if you don't do it right, you dramatically raise the risk of injuring yourself, not to mention that you will never get all the benefits that you can get out of your regime.

Once you have a weight guru, though, remember that you're the one who's in charge, so only do what you like, at your own speed and pace, trying to make incremental increases that are reasonable. I have suffered injuries—and not just to my ego—from trying to lift too much too quickly. So take your time in getting stronger.

Finally, I must mention one specific drawback to weight training, mainly because my wife keeps calling me a weight-lifting bulimic (it's not that I do a set of weights, vomit, do another set, vomit again, etc.; it's only her inaccurate term to imply that I'm trying to resistance-train too much): infatuation with muscle growth can be addictive. That is, one can do too much weight training, and this is especially true, studies have shown, for men, who can become obsessed with "bulking up" and sometimes risk using steroids to do so. I've never used steroids, by the way— I've suffered enough "roid rage" in my life from hemmorhoids acting up.

Get Flexible: A Stretch in Time Saves Whines

To be honest, I don't have much to say about flexibility, which is defined as a joint's ability to move through a full range of motion, not because I don't actually have opinions on the topic—I'm a Jewish male, after all, so I even have an opinion about crossing a street—but rather, it's that there just isn't much information available about the health benefits—or lack of same—of stretching and flexibility.

What studies we do have indicate that, as noted earlier, pre-exercise stretching does not seem to prevent injuries such as back pain, and the studies about stretching reducing post-muscle soreness show at best a minimal effect. Flexibility, however, is important for seniors. It probably helps lower the risk of falls and certainly improves seniors' abilities to do lots of normal daily activities that we younger folks take for granted (reaching for something you dropped, turning to talk to someone, etc.) but that become much harder to manage as we age and lose our flexibility. There is also this to be said for flexiblility: the kinds of practices that focus on stretching and flexibility as major components—yoga, Pilates, ballet, dance, etc.—have many other health benefits. Besides, stretching just feels so damn good (a good post-exercise stretching regime is often a great reward for sticking to a workout).

So given that I can't really see any downside to stretching and becoming more flexible ("Better take a break from this activity, Hister, you're just too flexible"; I don't think so), you ought to work on stretching as part of an all-around fitness regime.

There are several kinds of stretches (isometric, dynamic, and others), but for most of us, static stretches—which involve no motion (just think of me watching Manchester United on the tube)—are the ones to start with. In a static stretch, you stretch as far as you can comfortably go and you hold it. How long do you hold the stretch? Truth is, no one really knows, but it's generally agreed that 30 seconds or so is probably a good time to aim for. Is 60 seconds sometimes better? I told you, no one knows.

Here's another one: are there right ways and wrong ways to stretch? Yes, or at least there is nearly always a less good way (meaning, for example, that if you don't keep your hips at a certain angle to your torso, you don't get as many of the benefits of certain stretches as you would if you kept your hips at the proper angle). It's a good idea to look up on the Net the instructions for the particular stretches you want to do or even better, buy a book on stretching, which will invariably contain delightful photographs of people in positions you probably won't manage to get into even in your next life.

One final thing. There is consensus on at least one issue: everyone agrees that it's best to stretch muscles that are already warmed up, so don't do as I see so many runners doing in races (when they think someone is observing them) and stretch dramatically just before the race starts.

Remember this good-life rule: first the underpants, then the pants. So, first a light warm-up jog to get the muscles working, and then the stretching.

Get Some Balance in Your Life

I had no idea how much my balance had deteriorated until I started exercise classes with those young trainers. They are all able to rock on an exercise ball or on a balancer for hours at a time, whereas I got on and immediately fell off, I got on again and immediately fell off again, and on and on, all the time smiling like an idiot to indicate that this wasn't really bothering me even though I was crying inside. Eventually, however, with lots of practice, I was able to get to where I now go an entire two minutes without falling off—depending on lots of outside factors, though, such as whether the moon is in the seventh house. But when it is, hey, I can sit on a ball, and if you think that's no big deal, you try it, big boy. Be prepared to smile like an idiot, though.

Balance deteriorates with age, as well as with certain injuries (especially to the knee). But you usually don't know it until you have some sort of fall or accident. Balance is crucial in maintaining proper posture and improving performance in many types of exercise. It's obvious, for example, that you need good balance if you're a cyclist, but I'll bet you've never considered that you also need good balance if you run. Good balance is also crucial for certain vacations. You have no idea how often Phyllis and I nearly fell off log bridges up to 9 meters (30 feet) high on the West Coast Trail while younger trekkers just ran over them. Balance is also essential in preventing injuries, especially in seniors, who are likely to have reduced vision, touch, and hearing, and who are thus prone to falling and fracturing their hips, vertebrae, and even skulls.

So you have to work on your balance as part of an exercise program, and the good news is that it's not that hard to reawaken it.

It's very easy to start doing balance exercises. Just stand in a "stork" stance, on one leg, first with eyes open and then, as you improve, with eyes closed. Once you get good at being a stork (no delivery charge), you can progress to sitting and then (whee!) kneeling on those huge balance balls, or to a balance board, or a wobble board. As you get the hang of it, I assure you'll soon have more balance in your life.

Sudden Death

Study after study confirms that the benefits of regular physical activity far outweigh the potential risks and negative consequences, but you should be aware of the latter.

To start, as stated earlier, exercise can kill you. Several studies have demonstrated that physical exertion of any sort raises the immediate risk of dying suddenly, particularly in previously sedentary people, especially men (although this doesn't really count, one person I know swears she nearly died the day her spouse decided to exercise for the first time since she'd known him). That risk stays high, by the way, for up to one hour after the sudden activity. Between 5 and 25 percent of all heart attacks are said to occur during exertion, though curiously, very few happen during sex—in large part, I suppose, because for most men, that doesn't count as exertion (or perhaps few surviving spouses are willing to admit how their old men died). Most sudden deaths during physical activity are due to previously undiagnosed heart disease.

The frightening thing is that significant heart disease can be present even in the very fit and seemingly healthy. For example, a male acquaintance of mine is the epitome of fitness—a nonsmoking, fiftyish, healthy-eating, lifelong long-distance runner with a normal cholesterol level—yet one day, while out on one of his frequent long runs, he felt some chest pain, which increased in intensity so that he was unable to ignore it. Consequently, he went to the local emergency room—he ran there, I believe—where they worked him up, and the following morning he had a quadruple bypass procedure. In other words, all that clean living had still left him with significant damage to his cardiac arteries, which hardly seems fair. He's back running, by the way.

There's also the notorious case of Jim Fixx, the original running guru, who died, very young, as every sloth is all too happy to point out, at the age of 52, which is premature by anyone's definition. But what many fail (or refuse) to acknowledge is that if he hadn't been such a running nut, he would probably have died much sooner (according to reports about his life, he had a significant family history of premature heart disease and outlived the other males in his family by 10 to 12 years; in addition, he himself had lived a very unhealthy lifestyle for many years before becoming an exercise convert).

So how high is the risk of sudden death during exercise? In the 12-year Physicians' Health Study of a group of guy doctors, researchers concluded that there was a "hazard period," which consisted of the time spent exercising plus about one hour afterward, during which the risk of sudden death was elevated by a factor of up to 45. That, as they say, is the bad news. The good news is that the overall risk of sudden death associated with vigorous activity was still very, very low, on the order of about one sudden death per 1.5 million episodes of vigorous activity. In other words, you have the same chance of dying during vigorous exercise as Osama bin Laden has of becoming the next George W. Bush son-in-law. But here's the best news of all, folks: even that tiny risk of sudden death from physical exertion is significantly reduced in men who participate routinely in vigorous activity. So, if you want to protect yourself from dying suddenly during a basketball game, say, or heavens, even during intercourse, start doing exercise, and keep doing it routinely.

Bone Problems

Moving on to another potential drawback of exercise, a recent study found that women who regularly ran very long distances (most of them were marathoners and half-marathoners) tended to have thinner bones than women who didn't run as much. The researchers believe that these women had thinner bones not because of their running, however, but because they were generally skinnier and probably did not eat as well as less active women. (They may have had hormonal abnormalities, as well.) A British Columbia study of male runners who had all been running for over 20 years (a long time to run without resting, I think, but that's the way we are out here) found that men who ran more than 96 kilometers (60 miles) per week also had thinner bones and lower serum testosterone levels than men who ran less.

Also, hip and knee replacement surgeries have increased dramatically among baby boomers, and one reason is undoubtedly the wear
and tear from too-vigorous exercise. At first glance, you would say that
this is an affirmation that "none of us were meant to run, so I think I'll
pass on that next 8 kilometers (5 miles), but not the nachos, thank you
very much." I think, however, that this has more to do with baby
boomers running very long distances (even marathons, for crying out
loud), distances that are unnecessary for health and may even be
linked to increased joint and tissue damage. Also, there are clearly
many people who are not built to engage in "pounding" sports such as
running and basketball, especially those who regularly experience pain
and inflammation during such activities or those who have physical
malformations (such as a discrepancy in leg length). Baby boomers
raised on a mantra of "no pain, no gain," however, have often persevered with potentially damaging activities and many of them are now
paying the price. But regular runners who don't have injuries or malformations have less joint disease and better bones than do
nonrunners.

Problems with Specific Sports

Specific sports carry their own risks, of course. Running in smog-
plagued, dog-cursed Paris is the most hazardous thing you can do in
that city, besides arguing with a waiter in a bistro, so if you have to exercise in Paris, I suggest you rent a bike.

Speaking of bikes, cycling is a sport associated with several risks. As
stated earlier, in men, frequent mountain biking has been connected
to reduced fertility, and recreational biking has been linked to increased risks of impotence and other urological problems in both
women and men. As well, one study of bicycle-related deaths found
that over one-third of fatally injured cyclists had elevated blood-alcohol
readings. So never drink and bike. And for God's sake, always wear a
helmet when cycling.

Any sport requiring twisting or jumping or sudden starting and stopping—tennis, squash, basketball, recreational football, soccer, and so
on—can result in injuries to the ankle and foot (including tears of the
Achilles tendon) and to the knee (including severe ligament tears).

Since those are great sports to participate in (they provide good work-outs and good hand-eye-coordination training, they're social, they lower stress levels—except when you have to yell at the ref or the other play-ers), the key with any activity is to always remember your age because, as my wife keeps reminding me in other circumstances, you simply can't do at 60 what you did at 30. And she's right, dammit, so you ignore that limitation at your peril. But, alas, that's exactly what a lot of aging boomers do, and the rate of sports injuries in baby boomers is climbing rapidly (most commonly, one study found, from cycling, running, ski-ing, and in-line skating). So hey, be careful out there and always act your age. No boomer should ever be seen in-line skating, nor should any male boomer ever wear a ponytail, put on a bikini, or rap along with Eminem. These things are just not in God's plans, and it's danger-ous to mess with that.

Always remember your gender, too. Certain severe ligament in-juries to the knee are up to 10 times as common in females, so if you're a woman involved in a sport where you can tear your knee ligaments, make sure to work on your balance skills, as well.

Then there's golf. As I said earlier, I don't consider golf to be a sport, but lots of otherwise sensible people do. So among the injuries and dis-abilities golf can lead to, there's (most prominently) brain shrinkage, which manifests itself with the urge to take golf "vacations" (dragging yourself from one set of 18 holes to another identical set is a vacation?), and the need to discuss all the golf courses one has ever visited with anyone within earshot, as well as less serious things like muscle and soft tissue problems, such as low back pain. Or as one physical therapy ex-pert told Canada's National Post, "The longer you play golf, the more low back pain you will have. Your body was never designed to swing and rotate a golf club," something that's pretty obvious when you watch the average civilian duffer trying to play this game.

One last specific sport to note is skiing (and its cousin, snowboard-ing). If you're over 40 and you continue to ski or—horrors—take up snowboarding, I am willing to bet my future earnings that you will suffer at least one torn ligament, or a concussion, or a fracture (or all three) be-cause the odds are simply against you in these times of 14-year-old, 2-meter (6-foot-6-inch) boarders to whom you are merely another mogul. If, however, you choose to ski, anyway, then at the very least wear a helmet and put on sunscreen (studies have found that you get as much sun on a sunny day while skiing as you do on a beach in the summer).

Overtraining

Although this drawback of exercise is unlikely to apply to most of my readers, I must still caution you not to overtrain. Clues that you are overtraining include:

- Chronic fatigue with exercise
- Poor performance despite harder training
- Muscle pain persisting for two to three days after a workout
- Lack of desire to train (though this is certainly not always just a sign of overtraining)
- Irritability (ditto!)
- Occurrence of repeated infections or mononucleosis
- Altered sleep patterns
- Altered bowel habits

Summary

If you've been sufficiently moved by my arguments to start doing more exercise:

- Evaluate your needs.
- Decide whether you need a medical assessment before commencing your activity.
- Honestly assess your time and availability.
- Pick an activity you might actually enjoy.
- Inject yourself with a healthy dose of motivation.
- Find a buddy to work out with.
- Get the right equipment for your activity, especially a good pair of shoes (though you can scratch that bit of advice if you've chosen to take up swimming; in that case, buy a good pair of trunks, but please, no Speedos on men).
- Set aside enough time to do your activity regularly and for long enough each outing.
- Start low, but not so low that you aren't actually moving.
- Go slow, but not so slow that you aren't making any progress.

- Exercise most days of the week (four to six), and if there are weeks when you can't do that—your mother has suddenly shown up, for example, and she can't understand why you aren't spending every spare minute with her—then go back to that "most days of the week" routine as soon as you can. (Exercising every day of the week is too much for most of us and will inevitably lead to burnout or an injury.)
- Start with aerobic activity.
- Add resistance training.
- And flexibility exercises.
- And balance exercises.
- Be honest with yourself and persevere on "off" days (hey, we all have lots of days when we don't want to, can't, don't feel like it, aren't able to, etc., etc., but you can get over most of those reasons if you really want to).
- Vary your routine.
- Constantly evaluate your progress, and if you're not enjoying what you're doing or you can't see any results, reassess your choice of exercise.

One final note: in this chapter, I've focused on running, walking, and cycling, and I haven't spent much time on other activities that are worthwhile and that are pursued by armies of you: Pilates, yoga, dance, and so on. You might think, therefore, that I am dismissive of such activities. Nothing could be further from the truth. Anything you choose to do that gets you more active has some health benefit associated with it, and although some activities—running and walking—offer greater aerobic benefits than others—yoga and Pilates—the latter offer greater gains in flexibility and perhaps even in stress reduction. So if that's what you're seeking, by all means go and get mellow before getting more aerobically fit. The bottom line is I don't care what you choose to do as long as you pick something that will offer you health benefits for your most pressing needs. And most important, make it an activity you will stick with.

And good luck! Send me before-and-after snaps, if you like—they'll go in my next book.

◆ ——————————————————————————— ◆

DR. ART'S 10-WEEK EXERCISE PLAN

For those of you who would like some help in getting started, here is Dr. Art's 10-Week Exercise Plan. This plan is based on three assumptions:

1) You are doing nothing right now (or very little).
2) You want to get to a respectable level of fitness, but you want to get there slowly.
3) You're willing to start with walking as the first fitness activity you pursue (swimming can come later, much, much later, and will be done without my help, too).

WEEK 1

- Decide whether you need a medical evaluation before you begin.
- Get that check-up, if you need it, ASAP (at the very least, before this prep week is over).
- Honestly assess your time and availability, and come up with a reasonable plan.
- Inject yourself with a healthy dose of motivation.
- Find a buddy to walk with.
- Get a good pair of shoes and some good socks.
- Set aside enough time to do your activity regularly and for long enough stints.
- Try walking 1 or even 2 miles at whatever pace you can manage. (I always do my exercise program in nonmetric measurements, but for those of you who prefer metric, that's 1.6 or even 3.2 kilometers.)

That's it for now. Not too hard, eh? Most of it, lucky you, can be done from a sitting or prone position. But get ready, because the work starts next week.

WEEK 2

OK. Are you prepared? Well, you better be, because today is the first day of the rest of your fit-filled life. You are about to take the first hesitant steps on the road to fitness.

You will walk 1 mile at a pace of about 20 to 25 minutes per mile two to three times this week. That should be manageable for nearly everyone, and if it's not, then do it at whatever pace you can manage. But I want you to do 1 mile each time. You can do it outside, in a mall, or on a treadmill. And it's even OK with me if you walk downhill (though I'd prefer you mixed in a bit of incline, too). And I repeat: I don't really care about the pace, and you shouldn't, either. Just do it at a pace that's brisk enough to feel that you're walking and not just ambling. And that's it. The hard part is actually fulfilling your commitment to do the time. But hey, I'm a patient man, so I'm willing to wait for you.

WEEK 3

Now how was the last week? C'mon, be honest. I'll bet it wasn't bad at all.

OK. For the next week, we will work on increasing distance and time. (If you didn't do the whole mile three times last week, take another week to get to this stage because I want you to do 1 mile regularly at least three times a week before proceeding.)

This week we move up to 1.5 miles (2.4 kilometers) four days a week. (The mavens of movement always claim that you should never increase your exercise output by more than 10 percent a week, and this increase is slightly higher, but I think that caution is meant to apply much more to those times when you're actually working hard at getting fit, that is, when there's a good chance of getting an overuse injury by doing too much, too soon.) Try to increase the pace, too, though that's not nearly as important as sticking to the schedule. The 1.5 miles should take you about 30 minutes, so you're at least partly home, because I'm not going to ask you to spend much more time at it than that.

I will, however, ask you to work harder, but that's for later. For now, stick with this: 30 minutes four times a week, and try to get in at least 1.5 miles.

WEEK 4

By now exercise is part of your life, and you're feeling so, so good about yourself, as you should. If I were there right now, I'd be patting you on the back because you have no idea how many people haven't made it this far.

Before you get too squishy on me, though, I'm going to pull you down just a peg by telling you that, alas, it's time you started to work harder. You should now be doing a half-hour of easy walking four times a week. That's good, but remember that the harder you work, the greater the gain, so it's time to up your pace.

This week, you speed up to a brisker pace, say, about 17 to 18 minutes a mile or so (faster if it's easy for you) and you up the distance to 2 miles (3.2 kilometers) every time you're out.

Don't worry, you can do it. Do not spend any time with a stopwatch or taking your pulse or anything like that. The way you know that you've hit the desired level is that you should now be walking at a brisk pace, not a leisurely stroll pace. In other words, you should feel as if you're working a bit, though you should still be able to carry on a normal conversation with your running mate.

So remember, brisk walking for 2 miles four times a week.

WEEK 5

How you doing? I'll bet you're doing just fine. And I'll bet you're even beginning to enjoy this. If you're not, don't worry you will soon. Just stick with it.

You should now be doing a brisk 2-mile walk most days of the week. You can take pleasure in knowing that many people claim that this level of activity is enough to seriously reduce your risk of major illness. It also allows you to eat more (woo hoo!) and leads to better weight control, as long as you don't seriously up your food intake as a result of your extra energy expenditure.

Now you have some choices. You can stick with this pace, this distance, and this time spent doing aerobic exercise, and that's OK. It will definitely result in health gains. Or you can decide to get fitter by starting to up any of those parameters. If you decide on the latter, please bear in mind that you should increase the effort in small increments (remember the 10-percent rule cited earlier). You're not in a rush, after all, since you have the rest of your life left to live healthfully. So take your time getting more fit.

If you're up to it, start jogging. You can begin at a pace of about 12 to 13 minutes a mile, which is roughly the pace you see all those shufflers in the park running at. Start by doing that for about a half-mile or so—that is, for six to seven minutes—and then finish the day's exercise routine with your usual walking pace. If you can't do six minutes, do three instead, but try to do it again during the walk, if you can. Aim to get in at least a half-mile of jogging.

Next time out, try the same jogging distance again. If you can, add in another three- to five-minute run during the walk. **What you're aiming for is 1 mile jogging and 1 to 2 miles walking, and as I said earlier, there's no rush in getting there.** Also, if you feel any persistent pain or inflammation or discomfort, get it checked out.

If all this is still too difficult for you, there is another way to try to get there, and that's by doing a walk-run regime. You start the first day by walking 4.5 minutes, then running half a minute, and you repeat this six times.

A couple of days after that, you again do six repetitions of four minutes walking, one minute running; then two days later, do another six repetitions of 3.5 minutes walking and 1.5 minutes running; wait two more days, and do six repetitions of three minutes running and two walking, and so on, every two days until you get to six times all running. If at any point you feel you just can't make it to the next level, then go back to the level you were able to do without difficulty. But if you stick with it, within a few weeks (if my maths don't fail me) you should be running 30 minutes three to four times a week.

WEEK 6

OK, now that you feel great—all right, you feel better, at any rate, not to mention self-righteous, too, because you've managed to stick with this new aerobic program, more or less, for a few weeks—it's time to up the ante. You're about to play with the big boys.

So, what you're going to do today, or tomorrow at the latest, is run a bit faster and a bit longer, but only if you've been comfortable running the distance and speed you've been doing. And when I say "comfortable," I don't mean it should feel like a walk in the park. I mean you should feel you're making some kind of effort, but not so much of an effort that you're totally exhausted by it. So, yes, you should feel tired, but tired in a nice way.

If you are, it's time to step it up. That means doing a mile at a 10- to 11-minute pace, which means you are actually moving that tush. But you still, of course, have to finish your 2- to 3-mile excursion. If you can't do a whole mile at one time, then do a half-mile twice during your workout, but keep in mind that you still have to fill out your dance card with that 2- to 3-mile commitment. That will never go down, I'm afraid, so get used to it.

WEEK 7

Week 7 is what you might call a rest week, though it's not a week of rest. Resting doesn't take a week and comes only on the Sabbath.

What I mean by a rest week is that I don't want you to try to up your output this week. Rather, this is a week during which you consolidate your gains. I want you to get used to running a mile at about a 10- to 11-minute pace, and I don't want you to work at doing any more than that until that distance and pace are comfortable. It should not take most of you more than two weeks to adjust to that effort, but if it does take longer, so be it.

So continue running a mile or so over 10 minutes four times a week, with 2 miles of walking on those days, too.

WEEK 8

Well, time to start some real running. I know, I know, you are running, and running a mile four times a week is good. In fact, it's better than 99.9 percent of North Americans manage, so you should be pleased with yourself. Real running, however, involves more than that, so if you're ready—only if you're ready—it's time to add in some distance. (From now on, by the way, you can up the speed as you wish. Most people seem to get stuck at that pace of about 10 minutes per mile or so, probably because to go faster, you actually have to train, and most people don't have the capacity to train. And we do want to keep this fun.)

You start by adding in a half-mile every time out, for a total (I used my brother-in-law, the dean, to do this calculation) of 1.5 miles. You're to keep that up for the next two to three weeks.

WEEK 9

Another consolidation week (is that a chorus of "Yay" I just heard?). **Simply keep doing what you've been doing, though those of you chomping at the bit to do more can certainly do so, keeping that 10-percent rule in mind at all times.**

WEEK 10

This is the last week I'm going to encourage you. That may be either the best news you've read so far or the worst. Or maybe you just don't care (nahh! I can't believe that).

OK, **my final suggestion for you is this: it's time to get to at least 2 miles running most days of the week.** I think you're ready for it, but I'm not you. If you've progressed at the relatively relaxed rate I've suggested for you, and if you have no pain, you should be ready to run the kind of distance that gets you pretty close to the level most experts associate with excellent fitness (ultimately, of course, I want you to run 3 miles or so, four days a week, but that will come in time).

And no, I haven't forgotten about resistance training. You should start doing that, too, but first consolidate the running in your life. Once regular running is run-of-the-mill for you, then it will be time to work to further beautify that already beautiful body. Good luck!

3

Eating Properly

Your Mom Was Right (Partly)

An old-fashioned vegetable soup, without any enhancement, is a more powerful anticarcinogen than any known medicine.

JAMES DUKE, MD USDA

Food is an important part of a balanced diet.

FRAN LEBOWITZ, *Food for Thought and Vice Versa*

MY FATHER-IN-LAW was a man of few words, but on the rare occasions he deigned to comment on something, his meaning was never cryptic. On his first visit to the West Coast, I took him on what was supposed to be a prolonged tour of our spectacular seaside and mountain views. On the third stop, however, in the middle of one of my no-doubt stale observations about the beauty of the scenery, my father-in-law turned away from me and muttered, "Scenery, shmeenery." Then he got back into the car and slammed the door, thus bringing our tour to an abrupt and premature end.

My father-in-law's words pretty well express the way I feel about diet. I wanted to call this chapter "Eating, shmeeting," but my editor demurred with the observation that surely I must have some cogent things to say about what my readers should eat.

As usual, however, she's wrong. After thirtysome years of being a doctor and discussing nutrition matters with patients, listeners, viewers, and readers, I'm bloody certain I will have little effect on this area of your life and that sooner or later you're probably going to slam the book closed and say, "Diets, shmiets" or "Nutrition, shmutrition."

You see, "what should I eat?" is one of those questions for which no one, not even God, has *the* answer (other examples of such impossible questions are: Is Toronto or New York the real center of the universe? And what in the world did Jane Bennet and Mr. Bingley ever talk about?). Nearly everyone, however, has *an* answer, but that answer only satisfies (or applies to) a minority of people.

There is simply no magical one-size-fits-all formula to tell you what and how much you should eat. Everyone has different nutritional needs, and they are greatly affected by one's tastes, physical status, and even social status. That said, I can provide you with some general guidelines to help you determine what you need to eat, and I can also help you make sense of some of the multitude of conflicting claims being made these days about what you should eat and how much of it you should take in.

To get in the proper frame of mind, though, try doing what I just did. Since I am a method writer, I've just made myself a very nice spread. Sitting in front of me as I plunk away single-fingered on this injured keyboard is my constant double cappuccino, a large serving of yummy corn chips, accompanied, of course, by bowls of medium-hot salsa and guacamole (homemade with lots of lime juice and hot sauce), some cheese (I'm a nibbler), and a bunch of gluten-free crackers (I'm allergic to gluten)—I was feeling quite peckish. I forgot to bring along a napkin, but hey, I'm a midlife man, so who the hell needs a napkin, eh?

The Yogurt Lesson: Why Everything Is Not Always What It Seems

Quite a few years ago I read a news report from some intrepid reporter who had managed to travel to a largely inaccessible region somewhere in the Caucasus, a region whose name now undoubtedly ends with my brother's name, Stan, and who discovered that a large number of Stanians were living in good health to well over 90 years (many Stanian men, for example, were still happily procreating at an age when average North American men had been turned into compost for a couple of decades). Stanian longevity, many experts quickly chimed in, was clearly due to the unpasteurized goat's milk yogurt that yak-riding Stanians ate in great gobs every day, while Cadillac-driving Americans subsisted on steak and French fries.

As a result of the article, yogurt sales in North America skyrocketed briefly. However, subsequent analyses soon revealed at least two holes in the "yogurt equals long life" theory. First, that most aged Stanians were not nearly as old as the reporter had been led to believe they were.

"You mean, heavens, Art, they lied about their ages?" In a word, yes, though that's not surprising really when you consider that most Stanians probably had no idea how old they really were.

"How old is Yuri the Yak Kicker?"

"He was born in the year of the really big pogrom."

"So he's 110?"

"Yes."

But that's not all they lied about. As I remember from the eventual deconstruction of this story, Stanians also didn't eat nearly as much yogurt as we were led to believe they did. Many of them didn't even like yogurt.

Now, the point of all this is not to knock yogurt (I love yogurt) but to draw a few cautionary lessons:

- North Americans are desperately seeking a dietary remedy for that condition known as old age.
- When it comes to pushing items that may lead to better health, the simpler the explanation, the easier the sale.
- Marketing is everything.
- I should have bought yogurt futures.

Science Never Lies, Except When It Does

The moral of the yogurt saga: you should always take news and analysis about nutrition that you run across in the popular media with the proverbial large grain of salt. But then you should apply a healthy dose of skepticism to "scientific" sources of nutritional information, as well, because science is not nearly as objective as its practitioners would like you to believe. In many—perhaps most, perhaps even all—experiments and studies, there is ample room for unrecognized confounding factors and unintended bias, especially unconscious observer bias on the part of the scientist doing the experiment.

Take Schrödinger's cat. What that weird German Schrödinger propounded, and this is now accepted by most scientists, is that until an observer looks directly at a cat in a sealed box into which some poison has been added, that cat is both alive and dead at the same time. It's not half alive and half dead like me after a good workout, but both alive and dead (you may have to be a weird physicist with hair growing copiously out of your nose and ears to fully grasp how this works, but trust me, that's what it means). The observer determines if the cat is dead or alive only when he opens the box.

It's somewhat the same with most studies about diet. To a large extent, observers determine the outcomes because they have to "interpret" the data, as it's virtually impossible to do nutritional studies that meet the gold standard for medical research—that is, studies that are double blind, randomized, and placebo-controlled. In English this means that the best studies are set up to test a drug or a therapy against a placebo, that people entering the study are randomly assigned to either the placebo arm or the drug-taking arm, and that neither the experimenters nor the study participants know which group the patients have been assigned to. In other words, both the study subjects and the scientists are "blinded." But this is usually impossible in nutrition studies. You can't, for example, divide a bunch of kids into two groups and give one group lots of calcium and the other only placebo, without anyone knowing who's getting what, and wait many years to see what happens to those kids.

Thus, most nutritional and diet studies are observational studies; researchers observe groups of individuals and then try to detect the factors that led to the important differences in outcomes between those groups. Some of these are prospective studies (for which the researchers enter a whole bunch of people into the study and watch them over several years to see what happens to them), and some are retrospective (for which the researchers look at a large group of people with some illness—prostate cancer, for example—and then try to match those people against a group without the illness to see if they can come up with a single factor or several factors that differentiate the two groups, such as the amount of meat they ate, or their exposure to sunlight).

Clearly, in both kinds of studies (but especially in retrospective ones), there is lots of room for unconscious bias to insinuate itself, especially observer bias in the form of "interpretation," which often amounts to the same thing. (I mean, just think how differently my wife and I "interpret" some of life's issues, such as whether, if you wanted to torture some prisoner, you'd get better results by showing him *The Hours* or *Die Hard: With a Vengeance*. Actually, we both agree *The Hours* would work better.)

To a large extent, observer bias is what affected those experts who embraced hormone replacement therapy (HRT) for menopause (most researchers saw what they wanted to see), which eventually turned into the now notorious oops-we're-very-very-sorry-but-you-shoudn't-take-those-hormones fiasco, though the HRT case is not nearly as unusual as you'd think. There are lots of other instances of bias in the interpretation of studies that have unintentionally misled both doctors and the public, sometimes for decades, such as the long-held view that the upper (systolic) blood pressure measure is not nearly as important as the lower (diastolic) reading in identifying future health risks, whether or not breast self-examination reduces the risk of dying from breast cancer (a controversy that is still raging), or whether you can repress and regain memories.

By the way, it's not just scientists who make unintentional yet vital contributions in leading us into errors; so do study participants. After all, do you remember what you ate three weeks ago? Never mind that, do you remember what you ate this morning? Well, for some retrospective nutritional studies, that's what you have to do: you have to recall what you ate, in what proportions, and when you started eating that food going back several years, which is clearly a test few of us would be able to pass, not to mention that diet is variable and that people often alter how they eat and what they eat to fit a new time in their lives, and they often don't adequately recall such changes.

So keep this in mind at all times: although what you are about to read is a compilation of my undoubted wisdom, it's also a reflection of my strong observer bias.

For example, in choosing what I will report and advise, I have at least one obvious and overriding prejudice that I am completely conscious of: I believe that enjoying your food choices is as important as whether those foods are "good" for you. Thus, I will not spend a lot of time on a Canadian study that determined that a diet including lots of okra, eggplant, soy protein, oats, barley, and psyllium could cut cholesterol levels by a staggering 30 percent, which makes the diet as effective as the best cholesterol-lowering drugs. Even though the researchers insist that such a diet is very palatable, I know I couldn't stick to it. I mean, cold cuts from soy protein? Gimme a break. What Jewish boy would ever walk into Schwartz's deli and order a "smoked soy sandwich, lean"?

Certainly no one I know.

Eating Right: Med Fed

Before telling you about my favorite diet, though, let me lay my qualifications on the table. Phyllis and I are children of the sixties, man, so we lived in communes where we shared kitchens with, among others, fruitarians, macrobiotic dieters, meat-and-potato chauvinists, vegetarians, low-fat and low-cholesterol maniacs, fasters, people who drank only juice for weeks on end (or so they claimed), people who cleansed themselves regularly (you don't want to know), people who claimed to eat only things that were red or green or yellow, even someone who swore he ate only "ethically" correct foods, and we now have a daughter-in-law who's a strictly kosher vegetarian (but beautiful, talented, and smart as a whip; I hit the Jewish jackpot—my son married a lawyer). I know special diets, so take my word for it when I say that Southern (or Mediterranean) Europeans have clearly won the diet wars. (Strictly speaking, the French are not Mediterranean people except in the south, but I include them in this designation for reasons that will soon become clear.)

In my admittedly subjective view, the best diet you can possibly follow is a Mediterranean-style diet, though in truth there is no single

Mediterranean diet, since countries as diverse as Algeria and France, Israel and Syria, Turkey and Greece (notice a pattern, there, by the way?), Italy, Spain, and Portugal border the Mediterranean, and each of these countries is fiercely proud of its own unique cuisine. In Spain, for example, they make a religion of adding some sort of pig meat, especially ham, to anything they can throw it into; Italians are notorious for hating the French (but then, which Europeans don't?) and for forcing you to eat a plate of pasta before you can order anything else; and in France, they don't really care which of the courses you favor, as long as you eat *comme il faut* and finish with cheese. Eating dinner in Spain and Italy and Greece always includes being offered endless plates of delicious olives as appetizers, but that doesn't happen in France, where appetizers are more often the kinds of things only the French have names for and whose origins you really don't want to know. The French eat the most delicious frites with everything, while in Italy, they served the last strictly potato dish in 1864. And so on.

Yet all these cuisines emphasize a high intake of:

- Fruits and veggies (which provide high levels of antioxidants, vitamins, fiber, minerals, and other vital and healthful elements)
- Polyunsaturated fats and monounsaturated fats from nuts, avocados, olives, and fish (omega-3 fatty acids), which largely replace saturated fats and meat dishes
- Whole grains and legumes (beans, beans, good for the heart, the more you eat, the longer thou art)
- Moderate amounts of wine

The other common factor is a low but regular intake of dairy products in the form of cheese and (yes!) yogurt (save in France where they eat lots of cheese). The Mediterranean diet has many close relatives and clones with names such as the cumbersome "low saturated fat and higher polyunsaturated and monounsaturated fat diet," the "prudent diet," the "healthy diet," the "DASH diet," and others. My own form of this diet might be more accurately termed the Mediterranean-Middle-Eastern-Asian-French diet because hey, I can't live without my hummus, tzatziki, and sushi, but for reasons of brevity, I will refer to it simply as the Mediterranean diet, or the Med Fed diet.

Chez moi, we eat lots of veggies, fruits, beans, fish, olives, eggs, dried fruit, cheese, nuts, yogurt, berries, and similar "good-for-you" foods. Lest you come to the wrong conclusion, I hasten to assure you that we are not in the least bit abstemious, meaning that of course we attend synagogue on the High Holidays (some of them, anyway), but also meaning that we eat lots of corn chips accompanied by lots of dips, lots of rice and potato dishes (I make the best roast potatoes: the secret is onion salt), and one of us (who do you think?) even eats meat (including, heavens, hot dogs), and we also don't spare the treats such as ice cream, halvah, compote, and especially chocolate (well, it's loaded with antioxidants, after all).

We also dine out a lot (as a househusband, that's one of my favorite ways to feed the family), favoring Chinese, Middle Eastern, Greek, Japanese, Indian, and especially Thai restaurants (if you're ever in Vancouver, ask Montri at Montri's Thai Restaurant for that special fish dish he makes; you will never want to eat fish anywhere else again, guaranteed).

In short, we do not practice self-denial, though we do avoid the high-fat North American versions of many ethnic dishes, and we often ask that our dishes be prepared with healthier fat alternatives to what restaurants usually provide, something most eating establishments are quite happy to do for us.

But that's not how it always was. Only five years ago, both Phyllis and I ate the way we were brought up to eat, a European version of the Monthy Python "Spam" skit: meat, potatoes, meat, rice, meat, meat, potatoes, meat, potatoes, meat, and meat. Just as bad, we fried or roasted our food as much as possible in butter or shmaltz (shmaltz is rendered chicken fat, the most deviously delicious artery-clogging material yet devised by man, or more likely, by Jewish mother).

These days, however, our dishes are usually baked or broiled and, God knows, even poached from time to time. When we do fry, we use olive oil instead of shmaltz and butter; we dip bread in olive oil and balsamic vinegar instead of slopping butter or (yuck!) margarine on it; for breakfast, we always have lots of whole-grain choices on hand: breads, cereals, muffins, biscuits; for spreads, we use hummus mixed with olive oil (Israeli researchers maintain hummus is as rich in protein as meat), guacamole, baba ghanoush, and tzatziki; we eat fish at least twice a week, and I've learned to love it (the best meal I've ever eaten was a broiled halibut steak and fries in Port Renfrew the night we came out of the West Coast Trail, though I'm sure anything would've tasted great that night); we eat sushi as often as we can manage; and we always have a healthy supply of fruits and veggies and homemade trail mix (generally including raisins, peanuts, cashews, almonds, pumpkin seeds, and cranberries—if they're on sale, that is) on hand for snacks.

Because we eat well most of the time, we can also occasionally eat French fries, roast spuds, fried rice, cold cuts and organ meats (me, of course), and lots of other things that some experts will instantly scream are not good for us—and are *verboten* on most diets—but which we enjoy from time to time.

But enough about what I eat. Let me now feed you some of the evidence in favor of being fed Med:

- Several studies (including the Nurses' Health Study and the Health Professionals Study) have concluded that the more fruits and veggies you eat—a vital pillar of the Mediterranean diet—the lower your risk of heart disease and diabetes.
- A study from India, which is suffering rapidly increasing rates of heart disease as the population adopts more Western habits, found that following a Mediterranean diet significantly reduced the risk of heart attack and death in people who already had heart disease.
- A two-year study of Europeans found that those who followed a "healthy" diet had a 13 percent less chance of dying from any cause during the study than those who ate more poorly.
- Another study found that people with elevated cholesterol levels who used a cholesterol-lowering medication and who combined the drug with a Mediterranean diet had much better results than those who took the meds alone. Just as important, the diet mitigated some of the negative effects of taking the drugs.
- And finally, the two most impressive studies to me: first, the Lyons Diet Heart Study, which enrolled over 600 heart attack patients from Lyons, France, compared the effect of a standard low-fat diet on future heart attack risk with the effect of a Mediterranean diet. The study terminated early, however, because the Mediterranean diet was dramatically more effective than the standard low-fat diet at reducing

the risk of future heart attack. Even more impressive to me is the fact that most of the study subjects who had been put on the Mediterranean diet stuck with it long after the study was over. In other words, the Med Fed diet is not only healthier but also more palatable than a low-fat diet.

- And then there is the very recent study published in the *New England Journal of Medicine* that tracked more than 22,000 adults in Greece for four years and concluded that those people who ate a Mediterranean diet were significantly less likely to die of any cause over the four years. And the more strictly they followed such a diet, the lower their risk of death. So as the Mediterranean folks say, "Badda bing, badda bang, badda boom."

Why is this diet so effective? Well, it's pretty easy to see why a Mediterranean diet is good for the heart. It leads to:

- Better LDL levels. In just a few weeks, a group of New Zealand adults dramatically improved their cholesterol levels by replacing saturated fats with monounsaturated or polyunsaturated fats without reducing their total fat intake.
- Higher blood levels of antioxidants (see below).
- Lower blood pressure.
- Better arterial function.
- Lower markers of inflammation.
- Better insulin levels.
- Less abdominal fat. A small study from Johns Hopkins University found that people who follow a diet high in saturated fat have more abdominal fat than those who follow a diet higher in polyunsaturated fats, and you remember what that abdominal adipose tissue does for your heart, right? If not, go back two chapters.

But a Mediterranean diet is not only heart-healthy; it also has lots of other benefits, such as significantly lower risks of:

- Cancers. Overall, it's estimated that 30 percent of cancers (including the biggies of prostate cancer, breast cancer, and colon cancer) in the developed world may be partially the result of poor diet, especially a low intake of fruits and veggies and a high intake of saturated fats. In the Nurses' Health Study, for example, women who followed a "prudent" diet had about a 50 percent lower risk of colon cancer than women who followed a Western diet.

- Diabetes. Among a huge group of male health professionals, there was a 59 percent lower risk of diabetes in those who followed a healthy diet than in those who followed a typical Western diet.
- Alzheimer's disease. A study from Chicago found that people who ate large amounts of polyunsaturated and monounsaturated fats had a 70 percent lower risk of Alzheimer's than those who ate large amounts of saturated fats. (Other studies have not linked fat intake to higher risks of Alzheimer's disease, however.)
- Memory loss and age-related cognitive decline, often the first signs of dementia.
- Stroke.
- Pain in those who already have rheumatoid arthritis and perhaps even in the risk of developing such inflammatory conditions themselves.

Better weight control (see below on weight-loss diets) is also a significant benefit of following a Mediterranean diet. In a small study comparing a standard low-fat weight-loss diet with a moderate monounsaturated-fat, low-calorie diet, the moderate-fat people:

- Lost more weight.
- Were much more likely to stick to their diet over 18 months (in fact, the low-fat people gained back all their weight after about a year).
- Had much better BMIs (body-mass indexes, a measure of how fat or thin you are—see chapter 5).
- Had a much lower percentage of body fat.
- Enjoyed being on their diet much more than the low-fat folks did on theirs.

Finally, perhaps the most important reason for parents to eat better is that their kids develop their eating habits, so the better they eat, the greater the chance their kids will eat well, too.

But here's something that's probably bothering some of you: if legumes, fruits, veggies, nuts, omega-3 fatty acids, and seeds are such important elements of the Mediterranean diet, why not just become a vegetarian? That way you would get the most important elements of a Mediterranean diet without any of the potential risks of eating meat or any of the toxins in fish, never mind how much purer you would feel just by calling yourself a vegetarian (though an American survey found that some people who eat meat "at least" once a month still call themselves vegetarians—just looks better on the résumé, I suppose).

Well, I would never dissuade anyone from becoming a vegetarian, but it's not necessary or even preferable to go that far to get all the advantages available from a Mediterranean diet.

For a start, a diet with fish and meat in it is much less boring than one that excludes those foods. I know, I know, you really can make vegetarian dishes that are very interesting, and my wife and I do that, but I defy anyone to make a veggie stock that is anywhere near as good as a great chicken stock; it simply can't be done. And a nut burger will never rival a fat hamburger, so don't even try to raise that one. Besides, you have to work much harder at making veggie meals interesting than you do if you just permit yourself to add in an occasional nice piece of flanken or a choice rib steak or some tuna sashimi.

You also have to be much more careful to eat everything you need to eat when you're a vegetarian, especially if you turn into a vegan (which is not a small car made by Pontiac but rather a purer-than-pure vegetarian). Yes, you can certainly get all the necessary nutrients your body needs—vitamin B12, calcium, selenium, iron, and others—even with a vegan diet, but you do have to take much more time and exert much more effort to ensure that you are doing that. And hey, the less brain time spent on eating right, the more brain time you can reserve for settling the really important issues in life, such as if Angelina couldn't make it with Billy Bob, who in the world can she make it with?

Finally, there's this: it's just not normal to be a vegetarian. Most primitive societies eat lots of meat, in large part, I suppose, because you get much more bang for your buck from a buck than a banana. If we are programmed to store fat for potentially lean times, it would make sense that we are also programmed to prefer animal fats to beans. And don't forget that the huge human brain (in some humans, anyway) requires much energy to run, and the best source of energy is, of course, meat.

FRUITS AND VEGGIES: YOU'RE THE TOPS

So now let's take a look at some of the important foods in the Mediterranean diet. One of the pillars of this diet is fruits and veggies, because they're so damn good for you. A diet high in fruits and veggies:

- *Lowers the risk of cancer.* A study of over 5,000 Brits found that those who ate the most fruit in childhood had the lowest risk of dying of any form of cancer up to 60 years down the road. Other studies have linked high fruit and veggie consumption (or specific veggies, such as tomatoes, which, because they have seeds are really a fruit, of course, but hey, let's drop that for now) to lower risks of lung, oral, esophageal, stomach, bladder, colon, and prostate cancer (but not cancer of the breast).
- *Lowers the risks of heart disease and stroke.* This is a gimme; nearly every study—the Nurses' Health Study, the DASH diet study, the Health Professionals Study, and many more—that looks at what effect fruit and vegetable consumption has on cardiovascular health concludes that eating more fruits and veggies has a strong positive benefit on blood pressure, stroke risk, heart attack danger, and so on.
- *Helps prevent blood clots.* Grape juice, for example, not only is rich in the potent antioxidants known as flavonoids but also helps reduce the blood's ability to clot.
- *Lowers the risks of age-related macular degeneration and cataracts, common causes of blindness in the elderly.*
- *May also save you money.* A recent American study concluded that in their senior years, men who had had the highest intake of fruits and veggies in midlife had about $2,500 less in annual medical expenses than men who had eaten the least produce

But what exactly, you may wonder, do fruits and veggies have in them that makes them so magical? Everything:

- Vitamins
- Antioxidants

- Fiber
- Micronutrients such as potassium
- Salicylic acid

◆ ———————————————————————————— ◆

BERRIES, BERRIES, BERRIES

All fruits and veggies are great foods, but, if you pressed me, I would say that berries are best of all. Berries are great because they are delicious, easy to make into desserts, great with ice cream and yogurt, low in calories, high in fiber, and loaded with antioxidants.

What do berries do? Berry, berry good things:

- A study of Finnish men who ate lots of lingonberries, apparently a big favorite in Finland (but then they also like herring and ski-jumping), found that lingonberries can significantly lower risks of all sorts of cancers and heart disease because they contain lots of quercetin, a powerful antioxidant.
- If, however, you're not willing to move to Helsinki and change your name to Jyrki, berries such as cranberries and black currants also contain lots of quercetin (as do red onions, apples, red wine, black and green tea, beans, and citrus fruits).
- Blueberries are also said to be loaded with powerful antioxidants, especially resveratrol (an antioxidant also found in wine that many experts credit for wine's health-enhancing effects). Studies in both rats and humans have indicated that blueberries may help prevent mental decline with age (but only if you can remember to eat them).
- In rats, a daily diet of black raspberries had a significant protective effect against the development of esophageal cancer and colon cancer, though I ask you, do we really want to protect rats from cancer?
- Finally, of all the berries, cranberries are said to be laden with the greatest number of antioxidants. Cranberries have long been known to help prevent urinary tract infections, including those produced by antibiotic-resistant bacteria, and the tannins found in cranberries may also stop ulcers by lowering the ability of *Helicobacter pylori* to settle in the stomach. Perhaps best of all, a small study recently claimed that

cranberries can even lead to a nice rise in HDL. If you're looking for a
cheap, great hit of cranberries, here's what I do after a workout: I mix
pure cranberry juice (not that sugared stuff they try to peddle to you)
with small amounts of good-quality orange juice and a tall glass of water.
It's not too sweet, it's unbelievably healthy, and it makes even pure
water—which I loathe (what can I tell you? I have a lot of issues to deal
with)—palatable.

◆ ———————————————————————— ◆

An important reason that fruits and veggies are so healthful is because of
their high load of antioxidants (grains, tea, even chocolate and wine also
contain antioxidants, but fruits and veggies are especially loaded with
them). To understand why antioxidants have become the nutritional
equivalent of Robin Williams, that is, popular with everyone, you first
have to learn about free radicals, which are not the Baader-Meinhoff
Gang or Chicago Seven out of jail but the inevitable products of metabolic and oxidative processes in the body (even breathing produces free
radicals, for example). But like the Baader-Meinhoff Gang, free radicals
are also dangerous because they are very damaging to tissues, especially
the heart and brain. Free radicals are not only directly toxic to your cells,
they also promote the transformation of LDL cholesterol into an oxidized
form that is also directly injurious to tissues.

To fight those damaging free radicals, your body needs its own Men
in Black. There is some evidence that antioxidants fill part of that bill,
not only helping clean up free radicals but also minimizing the oxidation of LDL. For example:

- Rats put on diets with lots of antioxidants in the form of spinach
  were able to reverse some of the normal loss of learning that occurs
  with age.
- Dogs apparently learn better (they learn at all?) when fed a diet high
  in antioxidants (after antioxidants, I suppose that "Sit, Louie!" is
  often followed by "You sit, Arthur!").
- The antioxidant resveratrol, which is found in red wine, grapes, and
  blueberries, has been shown to protect against heart disease and
  Alzheimer's disease and perhaps even kill cancer cells, too.

But it's not a straightforward case of eat more antioxidants and you'll live forever. For example, men with lung cancer who took the powerful antioxidant beta-carotene in an attempt to slow their disease died more quickly than men who didn't take beta-carotene. A recent review in *The Lancet* concluded not only that supplementing with antioxidant vitamins such as beta-carotene, vitamin E, and vitamin A is not effective in reducing the risk of dying from cardiovascular disease, but also that supplementing with beta-carotene might even slightly increase that risk.

So yes, by all means, eat lots of fruits and veggies, but don't start eating foods—or taking supplements—just because they can supply you with some added antioxidants.

◆ ———————————————————————————————— ◆

CARING ABOUT CoQ10

CoQ10 is an enzyme also known as ubiquinone, because, well, it's all over the place—and especially in organs that require lots of energy, such as the heart, where it has an essential role in energy production.

The most common theory about CoQ10 is that it acts as an antioxidant (but then, what doesn't?) that helps free up vitamin E to do other duties. If you feel you need to take vitamin E, you should probably also take CoQ10 (though perhaps the best thing to do is to reexamine your feelings about the need to take vitamin E in the first place). This regimen is said to be especially effective when the heart is already in trouble, such as in heart failure (and other conditions in which the heart muscle is weaker), so some cardiologists now prescribe "that CoQ10 thing" to their patients with heart failure.

As always, however, some CoQ10 champions believe it's much more useful than in that simple application, so it has also been touted as beneficial in either treating or preventing:

- Normal aging (levels of CoQ10 fall with age, ergo, replace it and you shall stay young forever)
- Diabetes
- Parkinson's disease
- Immune disorders
- Cancer
- Even, God help us, gum disease

Trouble is, there is really very little known about CoQ10. We don't know what the normal blood levels should be, how best to replace it, how to get it to the tissues that may need it most, and so on.

So until someone comes along who can offer definitive evidence about CoQ10's benefits or even normal uses, I'd reserve use of this one for now. Besides, I'm guessing here, but I'll bet most of you are probably already taking so many other pills that you really don't need another one—or two—or three—to add to that mix.

Natural sources of CoQ10 include:

- Beef
- Meat
- Poultry
- Broccoli
- Liver
- Fish

◆ ────────────────────────────────────── ◆

FISH: HOLY MACKEREL AND SAINTLY SALMON

Fish save lives, especially oily fish, which contain omega-3 fatty acids (a type of polyunsaturated fat), which you can only get from your diet.

For example, overweight Eskimos (Inuit, in Canada) who eat traditional Eskimo foods—blubber, bubba—don't develop much heart disease and diabetes, in part because of that high omega-3 fat content in their daily fare. Thus, the American Heart Association now recommends eating at least two servings of omega-3-rich fish every week because they can:

- Lower the risk of blood clots.
- Lower blood pressure.
- Lower some bad fatty substances (especially triglycerides) in the blood (but probably not LDL).
- Raise HDL.
- Reduce the risk of abnormal heart rhythms and thus decrease the danger of sudden death.

- Keep heart arteries more flexible.
- Reduce inflammation.
- Lead to lower levels of a hormone (leptin) that raises appetite, so you might even feel fuller on finny fare.

In the Nurses' Health Study, women who ate lots of omega-3-rich fish had a significantly reduced risk of stroke compared with women who rarely ate fish. This was especially true for those women who didn't take ASA regularly. And the more fish these women ate, the lower their risk; women who ate fish at least five times a week had the lowest risk of stroke. Nurses who ate lots of fish also had lower risks of death from coronary disease and sudden death, which is thought to be caused most often by abnormalities in heart rhythm; both were lowered in direct proportion to the amount of fish these women ate. They also had lower risk of the complications that accompany diabetes. In fact, fish may be especially beneficial for female diabetics.

Over in the men's camp, it's much the same. In the Health Professionals Follow-Up Study, a high fish intake was also related to fewer strokes (surprisingly, though, there was no special protection from oil-rich fish), to lower risks of death from coronary disease and sudden death.

A diet rich in oily fish also seems to help:

- Lower the risk of dementia, including Alzheimer's disease. Elderly French people who eat fish at least once a week have a lower risk of dementia than those who rarely eat fish. (How can you tell if a Frenchman is demented? He's nice to you.)
- Relieve menstrual cramps. A study from beautiful, beautiful Copenhagen concluded that women with severe menstrual cramps can get significant relief from a combination of fish oil capsules and vitamin B12.
- Fight depression, especially when other therapies have not worked well. In one small study of depressed patients who were not responding to antidepressant medications, 60 percent of the subjects who got omega-3 supplements experienced an improvement in their conditions, as opposed to only 1 in 10 on placebo, and the anti-depressant effect kicked in within two weeks.

- Protect against ovarian cancer.
- Reduce the pain and inflammation of rheumatoid arthritis.
- Reduce the risk of age-related macular degeneration.
- Prevent and control asthma.
- Destroy some types of cancerous cells. A diet rich in fish has been linked to a lower risk of prostate cancer in Swedish men, for example, and in women, to a lower risk of uterine cancer.
- Relieve migraines.
- Relieve and possibly prevent auto-immune diseases such as lupus.
- Protect smokers from COPD (chronic obstructive pulmonary disease, or emphysema and chronic bronchitis).

Before you jump onto the slippery fish bandwagon, though, a word of caution. Fish is good, yes, but that doesn't mean you can sprinkle fish oil capsules over your rib steak and fries and get the same health benefit. The health advantages of fish come both from eating more fish and from the fact that the fish meals replace other foods.

Also, how you prepare the fish probably matters a lot. In the Cardiovascular Health Study, the people who ate fish sandwiches and other forms of fried fish ended up with more heart disease than nonfish eaters. It was only those who ate baked and broiled fish who got the health benefits.

And as always, all does not go swimmingly with all fish, and these days, certain fish—especially shark, swordfish, and mackerel—contain so much mercury that they should not be eaten often. Some health authorities advise pregnant women and young kids not to eat those fish at all because of the effects they might have on their unborn babies. As well, in theory, a high-fish diet can lead to a higher risk of bleeding in pregnant women, though I haven't seen any proof of that in real-life studies. (Always remember what Homer Simpson says about theories: "In theory, communism works.")

Fish especially rich in omega-3 fats are:

- Sardines (one of my friends says that an especially great way to eat sardines is to broil fresh sardines on the barbie, but then this guy also has a thing for horsemeat; how can anyone eat Trigger?)

- Tuna
- Mackerel
- Salmon
- Swordfish

Nonfish sources of omega-3 fatty acids include:

- Tofu
- Vegetable oils such as soybean and canola
- Walnuts
- Flaxseed

GRAINS: RYE YOU SHOULD WHEAT MORE BARLEY

Like fruits and veggies, grains are an excellent source of antioxidants and fiber. Many studies show that eating whole grains can also lower the risks of cancer, heart disease, and other diseases. In one study, Norwegians who ate the highest amounts of whole grain had a 23 percent lower risk of heart disease, and those who ate the highest amounts of whole grain also had a 21 percent lower risk of death from cancer.

Another recent study concluded that men who ate one serving of whole-grain cereal a day were 20 percent less likely to die of heart disease and had a 27 percent lower risk of death from any cause than their non-whole-grain-eating brothers, and the more whole-grain cereal consumed by these guys, the better their prognosis.

In my favorite study of all, *seniors* who added two slices of whole-grain bread to their diet every day experienced a subsequent 21 percent lower risk of heart attack. I love this study not only because it shows that it's never too late to make health changes in your life but also because the whole-grain bread these seniors added was in the form of pumpernickel, which, alas, I can no longer eat (because of my gluten allergy) but which still brings back such warm memories of my childhood (my dad was a bread jobber and I often helped him, and the reward I got for waking up at four on those cold Montreal mornings was part of the first fresh loaf of steaming bread as it came out of a brick oven—that, my friends, is as close to heaven as you can get).

◆ ────────────────────────────────── ◆

FIBER: THE LOW-DOWN ON GRAIN

Fiber is one food constituent that can be very hard to push, though anyone eating lots of fiber certainly doesn't have to push, heh, heh. What I mean is that fiber doesn't turn many of us on. If you are one of those rare people who gets excited at the sight of a bowl of oatmeal or a plate of celery, you can probably skip the rest of this paean to fiber. If, however, you are an average person, please read on, because this is important stuff.

There are two kinds of fiber: insoluble and soluble. Insoluble fiber (which includes lignans and cellulose) is found in:

- Many fruits and veggies
- Dried fruits
- Wheat bran
- Brown rice
- Whole-grain products
- Nuts (including peanut butter)
- Seeds

Insoluble fiber does not dissolve in water but rather attracts and holds on to water, so it makes your stool bulkier and softer, and as anyone who has ever had problems with harder or smaller stool can attest, you really do want softer and bulkier bowel movements. It's one of life's main goals, because if you don't consume enough insoluble fiber, you end up full of—well, in modern parlance, you end up fecally challenged.

Soluble fiber, which includes pectins, gums, and mucilages, is found in high amounts in:

- Oats
- Barley
- Beans
- Root veggies
- Peas
- Rye

- Nuts
- Fruits

And for celiacs like me, there is also soluble fiber in:

- Rice bran
- Corn

Soluble fiber is also crucial for proper functioning of the bowel because it delays the emptying of gastric contents from the stomach into the small bowel and beyond, and thus helps keep bowel transit time to a proper schedule.

Bottom line? The gut loves fiber, and so should you. If you eat enough fiber, you significantly lower your chances of suffering from all sorts of "Western society" afflictions of the intestinal tract such as appendicitis, diverticulosis, bowel cancer, and just as important for many of us, hemorrhoids, too.

In addition, fiber helps your heart by lowering total cholesterol and LDL levels. It may also decrease the blood's ability to clot and has been linked to lower blood pressure. And it may also help keep arteries more flexible and more open. Fiber also:

- Decreases blood glucose and insulin levels. In a study of young adults, fiber consumption was found to be a better predictor of insulin levels (as well as future weight gain) than was fat consumption.
- Helps control weight. One study found that men and women who ate lots of whole grains weighed about 3 kilograms (7 or 8 pounds) less than those who rarely ate such foods.
- Helps your brain (and not only in those people who have you-know-what for brains). After fasting overnight, individuals who were fed a modest amount of fiber did much better on memory tests than they did after waking up and drinking a sugar solution.
- Has a relatively low glycemic index. The glycemic index is a measure developed by University of Toronto researchers (blame it on Canada!) of how quickly a particular food is converted to glucose after it's eaten in a fasting state (particularly important information for diabetics), so the higher its glycemic index, the faster a food is converted to glucose (the standard is white bread, with a score of 100). In general, foods with a low glycemic index are preferable to foods with a high glycemic index, in part

because there is some evidence that the former leave you feeling more full and hence less likely to snack. This is not nearly as straightforward as it seems, however, since first, the index is based on eating that food alone and proteins and fats tend to affect how quickly carbohydrates convert to glucose, and second, many foods have a more complicated relationship to glucose and insulin production than this single measure would indicate (ice cream, for example, has a lower glycemic index than pumpernickel bread, but I doubt that too many of you would recommend snacking on a bowl of Cherry Garcia instead of a slice of delicious pumpernickel).

- Contains anticarcinogenic phytochemicals, which have been related to lower risks of cancers all over the digestive tract, including malignancies in the mouth, throat, stomach, and yes, the bowel, too. A recent review of over 500,000 individuals in 10 countries concluded that doubling the amount of fiber in the diet (either from cereal or from fruits and veggies) could halve the risk of bowel cancer. To be fair, several other well-publicized studies have shown that in people at high risk for colon polyps, a high-fiber diet did not prevent new polyps (most bowel cancers start out as precancerous changes in the bowel known as polyps, so if you can prevent polyps, you can prevent bowel cancer down the line). But if you ask me, folks, that's doing things ass backward, because once you're into middle age, it's probably too late to hope that fiber will do much about your risk of cancer. If you start eating properly after 40 or 50 years of eating the wrong stuff, a sudden gush of fiber isn't likely to turn that ship around very quickly. If, however, you start eating lots of fiber early in life—à la Mediterranean diet—then I'm sure fiber can and does prevent bowel cancer.

- Leads to better mental health. According to a study from Wales, high-fiber eaters tend to be less stressed and have better overall moods than nonfiber eaters (all that gas keeps the mood light, I suppose). But before you swallow that finding whole, I must caution you that it was funded by a well-known breakfast cereal company.

So add some fiber to your diet, folks. Not only will your tuchis be touched by it, the rest of you will be, too. A final word of warning, though: if you're going to start eating more fiber (actually, if you're going to add any fiber at all), please do so slowly, not only because the inevitable bloating and gas that follow can be uncomfortable to deal with for the first while, but also because you want to keep your friends. Can you spell borborygmi? Or diarrhea? Without spell-check, I mean.

◆ ———————————————————————————— ◆

LEGUMES: PEAS BE WITH YOU

I love legumes. About the only negative thing I can say about beans is that Hitler loved them, too, though no one apparently had the guts to tell him he ate too many. Well, would you have? Legumes:

- Have a high soluble fiber content
- Help reduce total cholesterol and LDL levels
- Improve insulin resistance
- Are relatively rich in potassium, calcium, and other minerals
- Are rich in folic acid
- Are relatively fat-free
- Fill you up

No wonder, then, that beans are so good for the heart. In one large study, men and women who ate beans at least four times a week had lower blood pressures, lower total cholesterol levels, and less diabetes over 19 years than those who ate beans only once a week or less often. Consequently, bean eaters also suffered 22 percent less heart disease, though big bean boffins also had to live in houses with *big, big* windows that opened wide.

NUTS: TO YOU

I am thrilled to note that the scientific world has finally caught up to me and developed a fondness for nuts—no, not the kind of nuts I used to associate with in my younger, left-wing days (Private Property Is Theft! Viva Che! Down with Everything!), but rather walnuts, pecans, almonds, and the rest of that nutty crew. You see, I've long eaten handfuls of nuts throughout the day, especially when we go canoeing or backpacking, since several types of nuts are an integral part of my outstanding homemade trail mix. A few handfuls of that and you can walk or paddle all day without needing between-meal snacks. And although it's true that nuts are loaded with calories, if you eat a reasonable amount, and especially if you use the nuts to replace other sources of fat in your diet, nuts might even help you control weight because they satisfy hunger and lead to less of a tendency to snack on less healthful foods.

Best of all, though, nuts are now known to be very good for you:

- According to the Nurses' Health Study, women who reported eating the equivalent of a handful of nuts or a tablespoon of peanut butter most days of the week had a 20 percent lower risk of developing Type 2 diabetes than non-nut-noshing nurses.
- Those nurses who ate nuts frequently also had a reduced rate of both fatal and nonfatal heart attacks.
- Almonds, peanuts, and peanut butter are great sources of boron, and a recent study found that men who consume the most boron are less likely to develop prostate cancer than their boron-bereft bros. So to pamper your prostate, guys, bore into the boron. (By the way, red wine is also a great source of boron, as is chocolate.)
- Rats that were bred to develop high blood pressure but that were given a diet high in a type of oil found in nuts (and fish) actually experienced a drop in their blood pressures and managed to retain their memory functions much longer than rats not given a similar diet.
- Researchers from France claim that the more walnuts you eat, the lower your cholesterol levels (though before you swallow that outright, it might interest you to learn that France has a very large walnut-growing industry—not that there's anything wrong with that).
- Six—count 'em, six—studies presented at the Federation of American Societies for Experimental Biology conference in 2002 (some of which were sponsored by the Almond Board of California, of course; ain't capitalism grand?) claimed that almonds are very effective at lowering LDL levels without leading to weight gain. According to one of these studies, the more almonds you eat, the better results you get, because almond skins (almonds have skins?) contain a sub-

stance that blocks your body from absorbing all the fat the almonds contain.

- Finally, a study from the Southern U.S. concluded that pecans are an excellent source of vitamin E, and they also contain 19 other vitamins and minerals. But consider the source, y'all.

What makes nuts so valuable is that they're rich sources of:

- Monounsaturated fats, which help lower blood levels of LDL
- Magnesium, copper, zinc, and other minerals
- Niacin
- Antioxidants (folic acid and vitamin E)
- Fiber
- Protein

And yes, I know that peanuts are not nuts but legumes, but hey, anyone who thinks trivia like that is important is also the kind of person who knows that Gordie Howe was born in Floral, Saskatchewan. Oops!

DAIRY PRODUCTS: IT ALWAYS GETS BACK TO YOGURT

Most experts have a tough time deciding whether or not dairy products are an integral part of a traditional Mediterranean diet, since the citizens of the countries generally included in what we take as "Mediterranean" countries have decidedly different habits when it comes to eating dairy products. Thus, in France, eating cheese with every large meal is a constitutional imperative whereas in Spain and Italy, cheese is eaten much more sparingly. Even in Crete, where you might think they add feta to everything, the truth is that they consume only small to moderate amounts of dairy products (mainly cheese and yogurt), which are always eaten in their full-fat dairy form.

The bottom line is that it's not at all clear what role dairy products play in leading to either better or worse health outcomes. They are loaded with calcium (to quote Homer Simpson, "That's good"), but the full-fat forms are also loaded with saturated fats ("That's bad"). They're high in protein ("That's good"), but they're also high in calories ("That's bad"). They have lots of minerals ("That's good"), but for many people who have a lactose intolerance, they are hard to digest ("Can I go now?").

So, I'm afraid that this is another of those issues about which you are going to have to make up your own mind. If you're wondering about me, though, I go with the French—partway, at any rate. I love cheese and yogurt, and I eat some of both daily (I generally eat lower-fat, never fat-free, yogurt), but I rarely eat—and never cook with—butter. I also drink skim milk, but only as part of my several daily cappuccinos.

Dairy products might help with:

- *Overall mortality.* As noted earlier, a recent study on Cretans found that a Mediterranean diet that included a small amount of dairy products eaten daily led to a significantly reduced risk of premature death. As well, in a 25-year study, a group of Scottish men who drank milk daily had a slightly lower risk of dying from any cause than did men who didn't, as my friend Jack does, order "Milk!" every time they dined.
- A *reduced risk of breast cancer.* In a huge study of postmenopausal Norwegian women, those who had consumed the most dairy products during childhood had the lowest subsequent risk of breast cancer, and it didn't matter if the dairy products were low-fat or not; all dairy products offered this protection.
- *Maintaining weight.* This is the one that might resonate the most with you. A study found that young kids who ate unlimited amounts of calcium-rich dairy products were the least likely to end up obese later (ding!). Another study, from Hawaii, found that young girls who consumed the most calcium from dairy products or supplements weighed less than their peers who consumed less calcium (ding!). Even better, in a two-year study of young women who didn't follow any special weight-control diet, those women who took extra calcium (average 1,000 mg/day) ended up being less fat than did their noncalcium-taking sisters (ding, ding, ding!). Interestingly, women who got their calcium from dairy products did better at controlling their weight than did women who got their calcium from other sources (leafy veggies, nuts, beans). Also, in another study, people who added yogurt to a low-cal diet lost more weight than those who followed a low-cal diet sans yogurt. Consider the source,

though: this study was funded by the fine folks who bring you Yoplait. This does not mean that dairy products and calcium are magic weight-loss aids; it just means that adhering to a full and varied diet with dairy products as a part of it is probably the best way to control your weight.

- *Insulin resistance and diabetes.* In a study of 3,000 young adults published in the *Journal of the American Medical Association,* overweight people who followed a diet rich in dairy products (including butter and cheese) were least likely to develop insulin resistance (and also most likely to be the leanest and to have the best cholesterol and blood pressure levels). The more dairy products these folks ate, the better their blood chemistry results, but it must also be acknowledged that those who ate the most dairy products were also the most likely to have the healthiest lifestyles overall.

WINE: L'CHAIM AND ALL THAT
Wine is also an integral part of a classical Mediterranean diet, and I, of course, endorse drinking moderate amounts of wine. To find out why, though, you'll have to wait till chapter 4.

Other Foods to Consider
Now that takes care of the basics of a Mediterranean diet. To eat right, though, and to vary your fare, there are lots of other foods you might consider indulging in.

SOY: SOY WHAT YOU WILL
Soy, what's holding you back from joining the millions of others who've leapt onto the soy bandwagon? Perhaps it's that you're smarter than the average bear and you actually look at what you're leaping into before jumping.

Soy and flaxseed are heavily promoted by food faddies because they are rich sources of:

- Protein
- Fiber
- Antioxidants
- Fatty acids (flaxseed is a good source of omega-3 fatty acids)

- Micronutrients
- Phyto-estrogens (plant-based estrogenlike compounds), which in soy are known as isoflavones, or flavonoids, and in flaxseed are known as lignans; both flavonoids and lignans are strong antioxidants

I know you all know where soy comes from, because everyone has had the experience of having to say to a new-age host, "No, thank you. Really. That soy burger was really great, honest, as was the tofu bun, and hey, what a surprise: tofu mustard! Wow! Wherever did you get that? But really, I'm just stuffed." But most of you are probably wondering about flaxseed, so let me tell you that it comes from the flax plant, which is a bloody useful piece of work because its seeds can be ground up to form flaxseed powder, while the plant produces fibers used to make sheets, so you can eat it and sleep on it at the same time.

So what do soy and flaxseed do for you? As a start, they:

- Improve cholesterol levels. A study from Toronto found that a diet high in soy (and other healthy stuff, including psyllium, which is also known as Metamucil, the powder loved by more bums than cheap wine) could cut cholesterol by nearly 30 percent. Flaxseed can also cut cholesterol levels but usually not as dramatically as soy does.
- Lower the risk of heart attack. A study of over 25,000 Finns found that those with the highest consumption of flavonoids had the lowest rate of heart attack.
- Lower the overall risk of premature death. A Japanese study concluded that men and women who ate the most soy were least likely to die from any cause over the seven years the study lasted.
- May lower blood pressure. A small group of women who were taught (coerced?) to eat soy nuts regularly saw a corresponding fall in their blood pressure levels of up to 10 percent.
- Keep arteries more flexible.
- May protect bones in older women. Postmenopausal Chinese and Japanese women who eat lots of flavonoid-rich foods generally have higher bone mineral densities than women who don't eat as much soy.
- May lower the risk of dementia and Alzheimer's disease. In one study, monkeys that ate flavonoids had much lower overall levels of

changes in brain chemistry that have been linked to the onset of a monkey form of Alzheimer's disease (a monkey with Alzheimer's knows what a banana is; he just doesn't know what to do with it). However, in one of those studies that leaves nonsoy eaters so smug, Japanese men living in Hawaii who ate soy were *more likely* to end up with dementia than those who had abandoned soy for a more typical American diet. One could argue, I suppose, that this doesn't prove anything, because people who love to eat tofu may be brain-damaged to begin with.

- May lower the risk of diabetes. A small group of diabetics who replaced much of the meat, eggs, and other proteins in their diet with soy products experienced a significant corresponding fall in their insulin and glucose levels.

In addition, flaxseed:

- May cut the risk of breast cancer. An American study found that consuming 5 to 10 grams of flax a day led to much lower levels of estrogen, which may in turn lead to a lower risk of breast cancer. In addition, Canadian researchers found that 50 grams of flaxseed rolled into muffins eaten once a day slowed tumor growth in women who already had breast cancer.
- May also block prostate cancer cells from growing as quickly as they normally do.

On the ever-present downside, however:

- Soy is present in far too many products that soy believers assure you taste exactly like meat but that in reality taste worse than my mother's boiled beef tongue *à l'orange*.
- Soy probably doesn't help much for symptoms of menopause (studies on this issue have been so mixed that one is forced to conclude that there can't be much of a positive effect, if there is any effect at all).
- Soy may lead to a higher risk of a severe allergy to peanuts. A study published in the *New England Journal of Medicine* linked the rising rate of peanut allergies to the much more common use these days of soy milk and other soy products in infants.

- A recent study found that male offspring of rats fed a diet rich with the flavonoid genistein while pregnant (genistein is present in high amounts in soy) subsequently experienced problems with sexual development, including larger prostate glands, and (yikes!) smaller testicles. I doubt that this is a big problem in humans, but until they debunk it fully, pregnant women might want to avoid eating too much soy—unless, of course, they would prefer sons with smaller testicles.

I know you all know this, but I have to include it, anyway. You can get soy from:

- Tofu
- Soy milk
- Soy protein products
- Boiled soybeans (yum, yum)
- Soy nuts
- Miso
- Soy flour
- Soy yogurt
- Soy drinks

MEAT: TURN UP THE MEAT

My regard for *viande* is like Woody Allen's feelings for Diane Keaton in *Annie Hall*: I lurf meat. I lurf meat so much that I can recall only one occasion—when Foxie's mother (this was in grade school and I was known as Hissy) served me boiled pancreas (at least I think she had boiled it)—in which my 100 percent record of instantly devouring every meat dish in front of me was ever threatened.

But the day my wife gave up meat ("I'm not eating that crap any more!" was her polite way of letting me know she didn't like the brisket) I realized that I didn't need to eat meat twice, and often three times, a day. As a result of her gentle prodding (she refused to eat with me if I kept eating meat), I have become an incomplete convert to her ways. Thus, I now eat meat perhaps once a week, and then only if I am wife-free for lunch or dinner. Otherwise, *chez nous*, dinner generally consists of fish or eggs or pasta and lots and lots and lots of veggies and beans (you might take that into account when considering dropping in unannounced after dinner). But I feel just as full and content after meals as I did when every dinner meant chicken or some cut of beef, with one huge added bonus: I never leave the table feeling too full. In my meat-eating days, I never learned to use my shut-off valve, so my meat portions were invariably large enough to feed at least three more Arties.

That still happens on occasion when we go out. I still remember my steak (it was actually half a cow) at a famous steak house in Phoenix last year. Afterward I kept threatening to divorce my wife because she had not only allowed me to eat it but laughed at me for feeling so uncomfortable later that night.

There's just something about meat that makes you eat too much of it—maybe it's the cost, or perhaps it's the bloody juices—but whatever it is, when you finish a meat meal, you often feel too full, that I-can't-believe-I-ate-the-whole-thing syndrome, which, curiously, very rarely happens when the main course consists of plaice or polenta or pasta. And you know what? I enjoy meatless meals just as much as I enjoyed meat-full meals. So, that's the first thing I want to stress in this section: you don't have to eat meat to enjoy your meals.

You also don't need to eat meat to have a nutritious diet. My mom used to wail that I needed to eat meat because it has so much protein, and "You need protein, Arthur, if you want to grow up big and strong like your father." Well, I grew up to be even bigger than my 1.57-meter (5-foot-2-inch) dad, but I didn't really need all that protein (I think I would have made it to this height without its help), and I especially didn't need to get it from meat.

Most North Americans eat an excess of protein, which may even be harmful. But much more to the point, protein is available from lots of meatless sources, including eggs, dairy products, fish, beans, nuts, seeds, and grains.

Now, if you love your T-bone and pork loin and brisket, I'm not about to tell you to give them up. As part of my wonderful Med Fed diet, you can eat meat, so long as you also eat lots of veggies and grains and fish. I will encourage you, though, to do two things. One, watch your meat portions, and two, leave meat out of some meals where you have come to automatically expect it. Also remember that all meat is not created equal; chicken and other poultry, for example, contain much higher amounts of unsaturated fats than beef.

That said, here are some negative findings associated with heavy meat intake:

- A higher risk of dying from all causes. A German study (and with 274 forms of wurst, the Germans certainly know their meat) that tracked the lives of 2,000 people found that those who ate little or no meat had about half the number of premature deaths as heavy meat eaters. Curiously, though, in this study (and hold your smirks, folks), vegans were nearly as badly off as the meat eaters; the healthiest people were either vegetarians or occasional meat eaters.
- Many cancers. A diet high in animal protein has been linked to higher rates of several cancers, such as cancers of the stomach, esophagus, and ovary and especially cancer of the colon. In one study, Chinese people living in Singapore who ate lots of red meat had about double the rate of colorectal cancer as people who ate little or no meat. But that higher risk was lowered, the researchers claim, if the high-meat diet was supplemented with lots of veggies. Similar results have been found in North Americans, though the Nurses' Health Study found no evidence that meat or fish consumption raises the risk of breast cancer.
- Higher rates of diabetes. High meat consumption has also been linked to higher rates of Type 2 diabetes, and replacing red meat in the diet with chicken probably helps control diabetes.
- Kidney problems. According to the Nurses' Health Study, people with mild kidney failure may experience more rapid decline in kidney function on a high-protein diet, especially if that protein comes from animal sources. Happily, a high-meat diet does not seem to harm normal kidneys.
- Raised homocysteine levels. Most homocysteine comes from the breakdown of meat proteins.

How you cook meat is also important. I eat grilled meat, roast meat, baked meat, and fried meat, and at my mother's, boiled meat. The experts claim, though, that broiling, grilling, and frying raise the carcinogenic content of the meat; however, you can apparently reduce your intake of those carcinogenic materials by picking lower-fat cuts, marinating the meat, and not eating the charred bits.

EGGS: EGGZACTLY

Eat lots of eggs (but not if you already have elevated cholesterol). I know, I know, most food authorities tell you that eggs contain so much cholesterol that you must limit yourself to one egg per day. That is a lot better than what they were telling you just a few short years ago, however, when they wanted you to eat fewer than three eggs a week. Happily, the eggheads have now rescinded that three-eggs-a-week-max advice because they've discovered that cholesterol in the diet doesn't contribute much to cholesterol levels in the blood, and besides, there are great individual differences in how we break down cholesterol. Some of us can handle loads of it; others have trouble with even small amounts. There is really no good readily available test to tell you which group you fall into, though most of us seem able to handle dietary sources of cholesterol relatively well (especially if we limit our intake of saturated fats).

So the experts now say you can eat up to one egg a day with no negative health consequences. But, you know, I'm more hard-boiled than those eggs-perts and I still think they don't really know what they're talking about. Since I love eggs and since eggs are loaded with all sorts of healthful nutrients (one study found that women who had eaten an egg a day as teenagers had a significantly lower risk of breast cancer later in life), and since eggs are the easiest food in the world to prepare (go on, tell me the last time you had an egg dish that didn't taste great), and since I've never seen a study showing that heavy egg eaters have any greater risk of any health problem, I figure that most of us can cheat a lot on that one-egg-a-day limit if we follow an otherwise healthy diet.

SUSHI: EEL YOU CAN EAT

Learn to love sushi (if you can get it) because:

- Eating sushi involves eating lots of different kinds of fish.
- You never leave a sushi bar saying, "I can't believe I ate the whole thing" quite the opposite, in fact.

- Sushi is lower in calories than many restaurant/ethnic meals.
- Sushi is cheap.
- Sushi is the quickest of quick takeouts.
- Sushi is not messy or greasy (not even the eels).
- Sushi is so civilized (if, that is, you can stomach eating all that previously slimy stuff that may not have been dead when they fed it to you and which has absolutely no equivalent in the cuisine of any other civilization).

One thing, though: never emulate a good friend of mine who eats at cheap all-you-can-eat sushi bars. There really is a noticeable difference in quality between low-cost, low-class sushi joints and better ones, and since this is raw fish you're scarfing, you really want to make sure it's of decent quality.

GARLIC: A STINKING ROSE BY ANY OTHER NAME IS STILL AS SWEET
Eat lots of garlic. Among other things, garlic has been said to:

- Lower cholesterol levels.
- Lower blood pressure.
- Prevent blood clots.
- Make arteries more flexible.
- Eradicate cancer.
- Fight infection.
- Ward off vampires.

None of these—except for the vampire effect—have been established in good studies, however. The real reason to eat garlic is that it makes everything except ice cream taste better.

CHOCOLATE: JUST DESSERTS
So that takes care of the basics—breakfast, lunch, dinner, and snacks—leaving only a couple of the elements of fine eating to be dealt with: dessert and after-dinner beverages. For dessert, what better treat can I offer you than chocolate—which is, unromantically, a mixture of cocoa paste, sugar, and both saturated fat (boo!) and unsaturated fats (whoo

hoo!). The good news, though, is that the saturated fat in chocolate is said to have a neutral effect on blood lipid levels, and I choose to believe that. Romantically—and I speak here only of making love to your taste buds—chocolate is a food of paradise, but it's also good for you.

Thus, one researcher found that adults who ate chocolate every day significantly improved their blood flow compared with adults who were dumb enough to get into the placebo arm of the study. He also declared that "the cocoa bean is among the most potent sources of flavonol," that powerful antioxidant. So eat chocolate, folks, because it's great for your heart (but remember that it's also chock-full of calories).

And if you have to choose, dark chocolate generally contains more flavonol than lighter chocolates, but why not have some of both every day, just to cover all your bases.

COFFEE: GOOD TO THE LAST DRIP

Because the health police were so down on coffee once, I used to drink coffee with much trepidation. But I dropped my trepidations a bunch of years ago, and I now drink my several daily double caps, only a bit of foam, untrepidatiously, because the health police, I'm thrilled to report, were all wrong.

The plain truth is that they still can't pin much on coffee, try as they might. Thus, the best studies have found that (with rare exceptions in very high risk individuals) coffee is absolutely not a risk for any of those health problems commonly ascribed by the health police as being linked to high coffee intake—heart attacks, abnormal cholesterol levels, strokes, and cancer. There are exceptions, however, so if you're pregnant or even thinking of getting pregnant, you should limit your intake of coffee to one to two cups a day, because higher intakes of coffee have been linked to higher rates of infertility, spontaneous abortion or miscarriage, and stillbirth.

For the nonpregnant drinker, coffee has a few other downsides:

- A study from Johns Hopkins University found that long-term use of coffee might lead to a small short-term rise in blood pressure (but no long-term effect, so if you have high blood pressure or a cardiac condition, it just makes sense not to imbibe much of what is, after all, a well-known stimulant).

- Coffee may increase homocysteine levels, especially if the coffee is not filtered.
- If you suffer from acid reflux or any type of dyspepsia, both caffeinated and decaf coffee often make the symptoms worse.
- Lots of people tell you that coffee gives them diarrhea, and they even make that sound like a bad thing. Hey, a faster bowel transit time is a good thing, folks, so I say drink hearty.
- Coffee intake has been linked to higher levels of rheumatoid arthritis. According to one small Israeli study, coffee might even hinder the ability of methotrexate, a commonly used anti-arthritis drug, to do its work.
- Coffee has also been implicated in higher levels of osteoporosis. Caffeine may lead to greater excretion of calcium and hence to greater bone loss, but you probably have to drink a great deal of coffee to suffer that effect. Besides, there is also some evidence that drinking extra milk with the coffee—say, as a café au lait—can counteract that bone-robbing effect.
- Some coffee drinkers do develop withdrawal symptoms if their normal, daily coffee intake is suddenly curtailed, though this certainly does not happen to every heavy coffee drinker. I often forgo coffee when we go backpacking, and I cannot recall a bad headache or mood disturbance or sudden spike in anxiety or any other withdrawal symptom on any of our trips. Then again, perhaps I'm not the best judge of that and the other family members might give you different version of what happens to me without coffee. Don't believe them, though.
- Coffee can interfere with sleep, not only because of its stimulant effect, but also because of its diuretic effect, which may—I can attest that it does—last up to 12 hours after you've taken a hit of the stuff. That's the reason I don't drink much coffee on backpacking trips, by the way. After all, the last thing you want to do is to zip your tent open to unzip your fly and confront that curious bear that is surely lurking by your still-warm campfire at 2 AM.

On the other hand, and many of you may find this hard to believe, drinking coffee has been associated with several health improvements, such as:

- Improved weight control, since caffeine slightly raises the metabolic rate.
- Lower risks of insulin resistance.
- Better outcomes after strokes. In what I consider the best study of the past five years, researchers determined that stroke victims might end up with less brain damage as a result of their stroke if they get a quick cocktail of caffeine and alcohol, dubbed "caffeinol." This doesn't mean, however, that if you're having a stroke, you should rush over to the pub to get an Irish coffee. These researchers used a special infusion that they gave the stroke victims by IV, though if your bartender is also a medic, then, I suppose...
- Possible protection against Alzheimer's disease. A small European study found a 60 percent lower risk of dementia in regular coffee drinkers, but I would argue that's largely because coffee drinkers are more likely to start with bigger and better brains in the first place.
- Better results in tasks requiring physical effort.
- Lower risk of gallstones.
- Better mental health. Yes, it's true, large studies have confirmed that coffee drinkers are much less likely (in some studies 50 percent less likely) to commit suicide than those who don't drink coffee.
- Better dental health because it has an antimicrobial effect.
- Lower risk of prostate cancer. Coffee contains boron, which might, as previously mentioned, help lower the risk of prostate cancer.
- Better ability to concentrate and pay attention (if you can get over the buzz, of course).
- Improved memory.

There is, however, one important confounding factor in nearly all studies done on coffee, and that is the manner in which the coffee is prepared. A much-cited study found that boiled coffee raises LDL, but passing the coffee through filter paper counteracts that effect by eliminating the coffee oils. Since you also eliminate the taste by doing that, why bother, eh? May as well drink tea instead.

And if you're thinking of switching to decaf, you might want to think again because one study found a higher risk of abnormal cholesterol levels only in coffee drinkers who drank decaf, which has also been linked to a higher risk of rheumatoid arthritis.

TEA: HEE

I have never been able to stomach tea because tea drinkers are just too damn mellow. Every Type B person I know drinks tea (or worse, soy beverages), and I hate them all because they're invariably the sort who end up just ahead of me in some express check-out line and chat nonchalantly with the clerk while they contentedly and slowly search for the 67 cents they need in their change purses. And the worst thing is, they'll probably all live longer than I will.

As an evaluator, however, I have to be objective, so I must report that tea has been linked to lots of good stuff:

- Tea is good for the heart because it contains antioxidants. Should you suffer a heart attack, one study found that you're more likely to survive longer after the heart attack if you're a tea drinker than if you're not. (And even if you don't, you probably won't care.)
- Green tea may help lower LDL levels (according to one small study), and it may also help arteries stay flexible.
- Green tea has been linked to lower risks of colon cancer, breast cancer, bladder cancer, and esophageal cancer, probably because of its antioxidants. One study in the *New England Journal of Medicine*, however, found no positive effect from tea on rates of stomach cancer, the most common cancer in Japan, where they certainly drink lots of tea.
- A study from Cleveland has linked substances in tea with a protective effect against skin cancer, though I'm afraid you'd have to slather tea all over yourself before going out in the sun—not really recommended by dermatologists yet.
- Still, another study found that drinking green tea relieves symptoms of eczema.
- According to a British study, green tea contains compounds that may block cartilage breakdown, and thus lower the risk of osteoarthritis.
- Tea drinkers may also be at lower risk of rheumatoid arthritis.
- Long-time Chinese tea drinkers from Taiwan have been shown to have stronger bones than nontea drinkers.
- Like coffee, tea might have a mitigating effect on brain damage following a stroke.

- Tea may boost the immune system by helping fight off infections, according to a study from Boston.

On the negative side:

- Tea has been linked to urinary incontinence (but I'll bet those tea drinkers are so laid back they don't mind leaking).
- Herbal tea may erode the enamel in teeth. (*National Examiner:* Camomile Causes Caries.)
- Being a tea drinker dramatically raises the odds of chatting in express lines while trying to find the proper change and thus causing everyone else in line to suffer a spike in blood pressure.

Doing It the French Way

So much for *what* to eat. But if you really want to eat healthy, it's also important you eat *right*, and when it comes to eating right, the French just do it better, a major reason, I suggest, for the famous French Paradox: the French do few of the things we suggest as vital for heart health, yet they have a lower incidence of coronary disease than North Americans do. Yes, it may be partly the wine, which is what most experts attribute the French Paradox to, but here are some other likely reasons:

- The French tend to shop every day for fresh produce, which not only tastes better but is probably more nutritious than canned or frozen or stored stuff (not to mention that fresh veggies don't require butter or sauces to hide their taste, as does three-day-old broccoli). Shopping daily also means getting out of the house and being more active and social, even if it's just to complain to the grocer.
- The French don't skip meals. Even if breakfast (see below) consists of just a croissant washed down with a café au lait (never made with skim milk, by the way, and always served in a bowl large enough to feed a malamute), breakfast is never skipped or even rushed.
- The French do not ask for seconds. During a meal in a French home, you might get eight or nine courses, but you reveal your low-class origins if you ask for a second helping of any of them.

- The French serve small portions, which is a good thing when you're serving eight or nine courses.
- Along with the meat or fish courses, the French also serve lots of veggies and legumes, items most North American cooks rarely add to the standard meat-and-potato-one-veg-and-may-I-be-excused dinner.
- The French don't eat between meals much. Aside from large cities like Paris, which functions as most other 24-hour cities do, though with far more attitude and far more light, it's nearly impossible to find restaurants that are open at 3 PM, the time of day when a real Frenchman — and Frenchwoman — does what real Frenchmen do in the middle of the afternoon (and which is also why the blinds on homes are always drawn at that hour). It's simply not *comme il faut* to eat much outside meal hours, although the French do snack on fruit.
- French meals are usually lingering affairs during which much family business is discussed and much stress is probably released. To the French, a meal is a time of pleasure, not an unavoidable and uncomfortable intermission between work and TV.
- The French also rarely feel guilty about what they eat. I have never seen a Frenchman or a Frenchwoman approach a dessert tray with trepidation, as most North Americans do, nor have I ever witnessed someone in Poitiers, say, or Nancy, take one or two nibbles of a slice of cheesecake and declare that they just can't take another bite because it's just too rich. In fact, they won't touch it unless it's rich. And yes, they double-dip regularly.
- And finally, they eat a lot of cheese. I don't know if you should eat as much cheese as the average French person does (see the dairy products section); France, after all, is a country with several hundred different kinds of cheese, and I think it's a loyal citizen's duty to eat each one of them at least once a year. But cheese is a wonderful treat, and, along with chocolate, it serves as a fantastic meal-end reward for having eaten so well during the main courses. And we all need our rewards.

Other Stuff to Munch On

Now on to some extra stuff that I believe is also very important when it comes to eating right:

1. Always eat breakfast. Countless studies have found that a good breakfast offers several important health advantages:

- It makes you smarter. Children and young adults who eat breakfast invariably do better on cognitive testing than do breakfast skippers. A study from Brigham Young University found that students who ate breakfast regularly had higher grade-point averages than students who spurned breakfast. At the other end of the age spectrum, a Canadian study found that seniors who ate breakfast did much better on memory tests than seniors who merely had water for breakfast.By the way, in case you want to see how well you would have done on those tests, three of the questions these seniors were asked were: (1) What color is the red line in hockey? (2) Who is the bigger moron: George Bush or Jean Chrétien? (3) If war breaks out between Australia and New Zealand, will the French surrender first? (The answers are at the end of the book.)
- It keeps your weight down. Data from Harvard University found that both men and women who ate a good breakfast (but not sugary, crummy cereals) were much less likely to end up obese than those who didn't eat breakfast, mostly because eating a good breakfast leads to less between-meal snacking and to less overeating at lunch or dinner.
- It lowers your risk of diabetes. The study cited above also found that breakfast eaters have less insulin resistance and, surprisingly, this held true even for people who ate unhealthy breakfasts. In other words, eating anything at all in the morning, even if it's a sugar-laden cereal, is probably better for you than eating nothing—though clearly a healthy whole-grain breakfast is better than an English fry-up of fried eggs, fried potatoes, and even—yikes!—fried bread.
- It can extend your life. In a study of a large group of male health professionals, men who regularly ate whole-grain breakfast cereals had a longer life expectancy, particularly from a reduced risk of dying from heart attacks and strokes, than men who didn't eat a healthy breakfast. The more whole grains these men ate for breakfast, the better they did (although surgeons and pilots should not eat too much in the way of whole grains first thing in the morning, given the close quarters they work in).

- It might make you happier. In a study of 127 people, those who ate breakfast reported being less depressed, having less stress in life, and smoking less than those who were regular breakfast skippers.
- It may bolster your immune system. In a study of 100 individuals, those who ate breakfast every day had fewer colds and cases of the flu than those who skipped breakfast. Just as important, even when they did get sick, breakfast eaters tended to have less severe infections.

  So your mom was right: eating breakfast is good for you. (She was wrong, however, about that underwear thing because, speaking as someone who has had to resuscitate victims of car accidents, I can tell you that we don't really pay much attention to your underwear when we're doing mouth-to-mouth on you. What matters much more, in fact, is what you've just eaten.)

2. Try to make sure that the food you eat is as fresh as possible, not because heat, light, and air destroy nutrients, which they do, but because fresh food just tastes better and you're much more likely to stick with any food program if the food you eat tastes good.

3. If, however, you really must eat canned or frozen foods (they're quicker to prepare, they're cheaper, and one study even implied that frozen veggies are more nutritious than out-of-season fresh veggies that have traveled many miles over weeks to get to your store and have thus lost most of their nutritional value), then try to find salt-free and sugar-free products. You get more than enough salt and sugar from other sources.

4. Take your time eating and chew your food well. According to a recent study, chewing your food well and eating slowly reduces GERD (gastro-esophageal reflux disease) symptoms (as may chewing gum a half-hour after meals).

5. Use moderation when eating. Don't waste too much energy counting calories or obsessing about how much you're eating (see below), but carefully consider the size of the food portions you choose. My wife tends to think she—and I—can be full on much smaller portions than I think I need to fill me up, so on the rare occasions she serves the dishes (we serve when we cook, so she doesn't serve often), I get much less on my plate than I usually take on my own.

And you know, that woman is right—those smaller portions usually are enough.

Studies show that when we are confronted with a surfeit of food, we tend to choose portion sizes that are larger than we need to feel satisfied. But we also finish whatever size portion we take. Researchers recently conducted an excellent study in a group of college students, who were offered varying portions of macaroni and cheese. The more free macaroni and cheese these eating machines were offered, the more they ate, yet they also reported that they felt no more full with the larger portions than they had been with the smaller ones.

Remember, you don't have to finish everything on your plate. Your mom was wrong about this one, too: that starving kid in China is not going to bed any less hungry because you failed to finish your meatloaf; anyway, these days that Chinese kid is probably eating more healthily than you are. Choosing proper food portions is especially important when eating out, so never eat in all-you-can-eat restaurants, and never be first in line at bar mitzvah buffets (if you wait a few minutes, the chopped liver and herring will invariably be gone).

6. If you feel peckish, you should snack, but only on small portions of stuff that's healthy. Eat only enough to take the edge off your peckishness. This practice ought to lead you to be satisfied with smaller portions at mealtime, and might help you live longer. A recent study found that even when they ate more fat, people who ate six times a day had lower LDL levels than those who ate only twice a day.

7. Read labels. If you really want to eat properly, you should at least know the names of the stuff that's in the foods you buy, and believe me, you're going to be amazed at some of what you've been consuming. Once you find that out, I'm also certain you're going to make some dietary changes.

8. If you're a parent, always keep in mind Jack Osbourne and Ozzie Osbourne and that thing about the acorn and the tree; to wit, your kids learn to eat the way you eat. Not only that, you can teach kids to eat poorly by making the dinner table a battleground. Remember, in the entire history of the human race, no one has ever beaten a kid

in a battle of wills over eating; the best you can hope for is a draw, and even that is rare.

9. I eat as much organic produce as I can afford, not because I think all those chemicals used in nonorganic farming are harmful to you (and besides, even organically raised produce has lots of chemicals in it), and not because I believe it's healthier (although a recent intriguing study concluded that organically raised produce had much higher content of flavonoids than nonorganically raised fruits and veggies grown in the same area) but because organic produce tastes better. I don't know how Safeway has managed to come up with a cardboard facsimile of a tomato that lasts six weeks and can occasionally be substituted for a baseball, but manage it they have, though that round red thing certainly doesn't taste at all the way I remember tomatoes tasting when I was a kid. Organic produce, however, does taste the way fruits and veggies are supposed to taste. If you can afford it, splurge on organic produce.

10. Don't sweat it about water. I drink only when I'm thirsty, and that seems to work fine for me. One study from Loma Linda University in California claimed to find a correlation between drinking lots of water and a lower risk of heart attack, but what else would you expect from flaky California? Otherwise, I know of absolutely no evidence that you need to drink the commonly recommended eight glasses of water a day. Nor do I know of any proof that drinking water is better for you than drinking any other thirst-quenching, nonsugared beverage, including coffee (a recent small study claimed that students who drink less than eight cups of water a day may be slightly dehydrated, but there was no way of verifying that slight dehydration leads to any sort of problems or that there was a benefit in drinking water instead of other fluids).

Besides, who needs lots of water if you follow a Mediterranean diet, as I'm sure you're going to do very soon, because eating lots of fruits and veggies provides you with huge volumes of fluids. I mean, every time I have a large bowl of a tomato-based vegetable soup for dinner, I also end up visiting the can several times that night. So my advice is to ignore the water police (you'll recognize some of them as retired tobacco *polizei*) and drink only when thirsty.

11. Don't use aspartame. (I hate aspartame, though perversely, I like Diet Coke, but as always, in moderation, which means only when accompanying a Chinese meal; Diet Coke should be compulsory with Chinese food). Whether it's ultimately found to be toxic or not, aspartame is surely never going to be found to be good for you.

12. If you have to sweeten foods, use honey. Honey contains antioxidants and keeps forever. I go to bed many nights kicking myself for having bought shares and shares of Enron when I could have bought jars and jars of honey instead.

13. Finally, I must address a food issue that Dr. Steven Bratman has termed "orthorexia nervosa": an obsession with eating right (accompanied by a disproportionate focus on the "bad news" nutrition items that liberally sprinkle daily press, radio, and TV reports).

    Take, for example, this thing called acrylamide. About two years ago, Swedish researchers published a very hyped study concluding that many foods we love to eat (such as baked and fried foods, especially potatoes) are loaded with a cancer-causing agent known as acrylamide, implying that we were all in danger of contracting cancer from eating foods we love. Turns out, though, on further research from the U.S., that acrylamide is probably not present in large enough amounts in most foods to cause harm to humans, and especially not enough to cause malignancies in the stomach and bowel (areas that would likely be most affected if acrylamide were indeed carcinogenic in humans). Further, acrylamide is present in many foods that are in fact good for you, such as breakfast cereals.

    Now, it may still be that acrylamide will turn out to be a bigger bogeyman than Yo Mama Osama, but chances are way better that it won't and that all that effort you spent trying to rid your diet of acrylamide would have been far better spent trying to rid your closet of outdated fashions.

    Never worry too much (or at all) about press reports of a new cancer-causing agent, because the press is paid to hype things out of all proportion. And never change your diet based on one or even two studies. Always wait for these studies to be confirmed—or more often, debunked—with further, larger investigations.

    Love my daily hit of acrylamide, by the way.

Summary

So, here's the key to eating right. Concentrate on eating way more:

- Fruits and veggies, preferably organic
- Whole grains
- Legumes
- Fish, especially salmon and tuna
- Monounsaturated fats
- Nuts

Lower your intake of:

- Saturated fats
- Trans fats (see chapter 4)
- Refined grain products
- Meat
- Prepared foods

Consider eating more:

- Soy
- Eggs
- Sushi
- Garlic
- Chocolate

Don't worry too much about:

- Coffee
- Tea
- Water

Focus on:

- Eating moderately
- Eating regularly: breakfast, lunch, and dinner
- Enjoying your food

Nutrients

You Really Are What You Eat

Tell me what you eat, and I shall tell you who you are.
JEAN-ANTHELME BRILLAT-SAVARIN, *The Physiology of Taste*

Nutrition... has been kicked around like a puppy that cannot take care of itself. Food faddists and crackpots have kicked it pretty cruelly...
ADELLE DAVIS

Y OU ARE WHAT YOU EAT.
Before I get into specific nutrients, here are a couple of disclaimers. In keeping with my aversion to numbers, except for a couple of exceptions such as calcium, I will not give you exact recommendations about the amount of anything you should eat (or avoid eating). Also, this list is not meant to be all-inclusive (I don't discuss zinc, for example, or phosphorus or iodine, or any of the other smaller-fry nutrients). I have concentrated on those food elements about which I feel I have something to say or that are much in the news.

First, I will talk about macronutrients, which you need in large doses—your protein, your carbohydrates, and your fats. Then I will talk about micronutrients, which you need in much smaller amounts—your vitamins and your minerals.

Protein: How to Grow Up Big and Strong

The less said about protein the better, because as opposed to what your mom used to tell you and probably still does, you really don't need to worry about protein much; nearly all of us get more than enough protein in our diets. Actually, protein led me to doubt many of the other things my mom told me (never go outside with wet hair, buy land and you'll never regret it, etc.) because I followed her advice and I ate a ton of protein as a kid and young adult—at least two meat meals a day—but I never made it past 1.68 meters (5 feet 6 inches), anyway.

Protein is composed of chains of amino acids, of which there are 22. The body can make 13 of these amino acids, but nine have to come from food sources. Complete proteins contain all 22 amino acids, whereas incomplete proteins are missing some amino acids.

Protein helps build, maintain, and repair body tissue, especially muscle. It also plays a key role in the production of enzymes, hormones, and antibodies and in the maintenance of the acid-base balance and fluid and electrolyte balance.

You get complete protein from:

- Meat
- Fish
- Dairy products
- Poultry
- Eggs

You get incomplete protein from:

- Beans
- Rice
- Legumes
- Nuts
- Seeds
- Grains

Thus, if you're a strict vegetarian, you need to combine protein sources to make sure you get all the necessary amino acids, though that really doesn't seem too difficult with all the options available.

CARBOHYDRATES: THE BODY'S CHEW-CHEW

Carbohydrates provide you with energy and also help you metabolize fat. There are two kinds of carbs: simple one (sugars) and complex ones (starches and fiber). Simple carbs give you quick energy because after digestion they convert rapidly to glucose, the source of energy for your tissues. Complex carbs take longer to convert to glucose, so they provide a steadier and slower source of energy.

FATS: PUFAS AND MUFAS, MOMMA

Despite the pejorative connotation attached to the word, fats are a good thing and are very necessary for survival. Among other functions, fats (including cholesterol):

- Are essential for the production of hormones
- Are vital in nerve-cell function
- Help carry fat-soluble vitamins
- Serve as a source of energy
- Protect organs
- Make foods more palatable

So it's not the fats themselves that pose a problem but rather the kind of fats you take in and the amount that can lead to health risks.

Saturated fats are straight chains of carbon and hydrogen that are dense enough to be solid at room temperature. Saturated fat, long the Darth Vader of the Western diet, raises blood cholesterol levels and causes the blood to become "stickier." A large intake of saturated fat has been implicated in much higher risks of heart attack, strokes, some cancers, and even Alzheimer's disease.

Your body makes saturated fats, but you get more of it in:

- Meat
- Dairy products: butter, cheese, cream, and milk (except skim milk)
- Chocolate
- Palm oil
- Coconut oil

Polyunsaturated fats (PUFAS) and monounsaturated fats are not as dense as saturated fats (they are "unsaturated," after all). Polyunsaturated fats are liquid at room temperature and are found in:

- Corn oil
- Safflower oil
- Soybeans
- Fish

Monounsaturated fats (MUFAS) are partially unsaturated fats. They are found in:

- Olives and olive oil
- Canola oil
- Peanut oil
- Nuts, including peanuts, almonds, cashews, and peanut butter
- Avocados

TRANS FATS

This is the one I want to focus on. I have a loyal listener to my radio show ("Go ahead, Ken from Coquitlam"), who years ago started writing me that I was a typical know-nothing physician (my loyal listeners don't necessarily agree with me nor even like me, for that matter, which makes them like family) who put far too much emphasis on eliminating saturated fats from the diet and not nearly enough on the negative aspects of something called trans fats—which, to be honest, I knew nothing about back then (Ken was clearly right about what I knew).

"Huh?" I wrote back to him several times, with my usual eloquence. "What the hell are trans fats?" Well, I soon learned more than I wanted to know about trans fats from "Go ahead, Ken from Coquitlam," and the more I learned, the more I agreed with him. Eventually, I bought into his program: trans fats are killers, and probably (Ken would say definitely) the worst fats of all.

Trans fats are those fats formed when vegetable oils are hardened, as in hard margarine and shortening, both of which are very widely used in manufacturing fast foods and processed foods. If, like me, you read food labels (since I'm allergic to gluten, which is found in wheat, rye, and barley, I read labels assiduously because you have no idea how often they hide those grains in foods), you will notice how prevalent trans fats are in your diet. They're that little thing called "hydrogenated vegetable oil," or "partially hydrogenated vegetable oil." Ugghh!

Trans fats are found in:

- Stick margarine
- Vegetable shortening
- Hydrogenated or partially hydrogenated vegetable oil
- Beef
- Pork
- Lamb
- Commercial baked goods: cookies, biscuits, bread
- Fast foods: burgers, fries

Trans fats do most of the things you really don't want food to do:

- Raise LDL levels.
- Raise triglyceride levels (as well as levels of other harmful fatty chemicals).
- Markedly lower HDL levels (which is why "Go ahead, Ken from Coquitlam" hates them much more than he hates saturated fats).
- Reduce arterial flexibility.
- Raise insulin resistance.

It is no surprise, then, that in the Nurses' Health Study, higher trans fat intake was linked to a substantially higher risk of heart disease: the more trans fats consumed, the higher the risk of heart disease. Part of the reason for this is that people who prefer to eat foods with trans fats in them also tend to eat less of the foods that contain unsaturated fats.

The Nurses' Health Study also found that incremental increases of as little as 2 percent in trans fat intake significantly raised the risk of Type 2 diabetes. However, there was no increased risk of diabetes from a higher intake of saturated fat or total fat in the diet (though a high intake of polyunsaturated fats lowered the risk of Type 2 diabetes).

"Enough with the fats, already," some of you are no doubt saying right now (though perhaps only those from Montreal, to whom *already* is the only adverb they know). "How does all this come to-gether?" Simple, really.

When it comes to the fat content of your diet, replace saturated fats and trans fats with polyunsaturated fats and monounsaturated fats. So:

- Eat less meat and more fish.
- Eat fewer fast foods and more nuts.
- Eat fewer commercially baked goods made with hydrogenated oil.
- Eat less butter and margarine and more olive oil.

In other words, you don't have to drastically lower the total fat content of your diet so much as change the sources of fat you consume. To that end, several studies, including the Nurses' Health Study, have shown that diets that substitute unsaturated for saturated fats (and trans fats):

- Can lower LDL levels as well as a low-fat diet can.
- Lead to lower levels of trigyclerides.
- Lower the blood's tendency to clot.
- Lower the risk of heart rhythm disturbances and hence lower the risk of sudden death.
- Lower blood pressure. One study even found that cooking only with sesame oil (which is rich in polyunsaturated and monounsaturated fat) led to rapid blood pressure control in a group of men and women who had previously been unable to control their blood pressure, even with medication.
- Lower the risk of insulin resistance and diabetes.

Researchers in the Nurses' Health Study have estimated that replacing as little as 2 percent of the calories in the average North American diet with polyunsaturated fats could lower the risk of diabetes by 40 percent. Other researchers have estimated that a similar reduction in trans fat could cut the rate of heart disease by 25 percent.

There is evidence in the real world that this actually works. The best example, I believe, comes from the residents of the magnificent island of Crete, who have among the world's lowest levels of heart disease while at the same time having a very high consumption of fat. Their se-cret is that they consume most of their fat as olive oil and as those beautiful, magnificent, stupendous, orgasmic olives, which they eat in Crete as appetizers, main courses, and surely even dessert.

And think about it: who looks happier in the usual pictures you see of them? The typical Dean Ornish very low-fat diet follower? Or the typical Cretan? I rest my case.

The Four Big Minerals

CALCIUM: SO MUCH TO DO ABOUT SO LITTLE—MAYBE

Most nutrition experts warn that our epidemic of osteoporosis and the subsequent high rate of fractures in our aging bones is in large part a result of our low intake of calcium (along with our sedentary lifestyles) and exhort us, therefore, to ingest a lot of calcium every day. Since most of us simply can't get that requisite intake of calcium from our diet alone (in part because of widespread lactose intolerance, in part because so many of us just don't like to drink milk or eat yogurt, tofu, and cheese), we are urged to take supplements instead.

But do we really need that much calcium? Calcium is certainly essential in our early years to help build up the healthiest possible skeleton. It's sort of like money—the more you start with, the harder it is to go broke. Similarly, the stronger your bones are to begin with (bones grow steadily until the age of 30 or so), the greater your eventual ability to deal with the inevitable bone loss that accompanies aging. And the feeling among most experts is that you can best maintain that healthy skeleton (bone is steadily resorbed as we grow older) by consuming lots of calcium throughout your life.

Currently, the daily intake recommendations from the U.S. National Academy of Sciences are:

- Children ages four to eight: 800 mg
- Teenagers: 1,300 mg
- Adults 20 to 50: 1,000 mg
- Adults 51 and up: 1,300 mg

But you know, I find it hard to believe that getting that amount of calcium into adults, especially by way of dairy products, is going to make a large difference in the rate of bone fractures in North America.

Although I'd certainly advise children and young adults (up to the age of 25 to 30 or so) to drink more milk (if they can tolerate it) to build up their bone mass, I'm not nearly as certain that older folks—especially those in the later stages of middle age and beyond—must do the same.

Why? First, because there is much more to bone strength—vitamin D intake, for starters, plus exercise, hormones, and exposure to sunlight—than calcium intake (countries with the largest calcium intake do not have the lowest rate of hip fracture) I believe that if we focus a disproportionate amount of attention on calcium (as we are doing), people are less likely to do some of the other things necessary to ensure healthy bones. Most people can focus on only one or perhaps two things at a time (especially husbands, of course). I'm convinced that the public, with its urgent desire to find an easy one-action or one-word answer to every problem (the key to Middle East peace is to deal with the *rootcauses* of local discontent, teenagers act out only because their *selfesteem* is low, pain ends when you get *closure,* etc.) has begun to believe that all they have to do to prevent fractures is to ingest more calcium, and this is simply *sillynonsense.* For example, most fractures in the elderly are the result of falls, and unless we do lots more to prevent falls—starting with, yes, getting seniors to do more weight-bearing exercise, as well as exercises to improve balance, and teaching them how to avoid falls in the first place—the rate of fractures will not fall (pardon me!) much, even if we get every senior ingesting so much calcium that she looks like a chalk pillar when she stands.

Also, as with so many other changes in lifestyle, too many of us only start to take these large recommended amounts of calcium at the age of 50 and beyond, which is probably too late to make a great difference in our overall risk of fracture, especially if that increased calcium intake is not wedded to an exercise regime and an increased intake of vitamin D.

Finally, there may be potential hazards from getting too much calcium, such as possible risks of prostate cancer in men and ovarian cancer in women.

Now that is not to say that you shouldn't drink milk and fortified orange juice, and that you shouldn't eat lots of spinach and almonds and salmon and maybe cheese. You should get lots of those things into you because they're good for you, and because they taste great. I have lots more trouble, however, advising you to take calcium supplements to get up to that magical number of milligrams you're supposed to reach every day.

If, however, you choose to disagree with me (don't worry about it; lots of people do) and you decide to supplement with calcium, anyway, please bear in mind the following considerations. To help your bones, calcium needs vitamin D (see below) as well as phosphorus, according to one key study, to get into your bloodstream and do what it's supposed to do.

Also, several factors can interfere with calcium absorption, including:

- A high-protein diet (a high-protein diet can leach calcium out of bones, too)
- A very high caffeine intake
- Smoking

For the calcium in calcium supplements to be fully absorbed, you probably should avoid taking them with meals. Also, a high intake of calcium supplements can interfere with the absorption of some of the other medications you may be taking and can compromise the absorption of other nutrients, such as iron. Theoretically, a high intake might even increase the risk of kidney stones (though that has been disputed in recent studies). Kidney stones are definitely one problem you want to avoid, however, no matter how small the danger, because if you want to know the real definition of pain, just spend a few minutes with someone trying to pass a kidney stone. The only thing that even comes remotely close to witnessing that kind of pain is spending time watching the New Jersey Devils play their brand of hockey, or having to sit through *The Hours* a second time.

Also, all forms of calcium supplements are not equal. Some studies have indicated that calcium citrate is more "bioavailable" than calcium carbonate, meaning that it's easier to get calcium from calcium citrate into your bloodstream, though other studies have disputed those findings.

Now that we've chewed on dem bones, a few words about some of the other potential health benefits of calcium:

- *Blood pressure.* Calcium might (slightly) impede the seemingly inevitable climb in blood pressure, especially the upper or systolic pressure, that occurs as we age. In people who already have high blood pressure, extra calcium might help their medications bring their pressure down.

- *Colon cancer.* In the Physicians' Health Study, male doctors who consumed the most calcium had a lower rate of colon cancer than their peers. In nondoctors, an American Cancer Society study found that calcium supplements (but not calcium from dietary sources) was linked to a slightly lower incidence of colon cancer in both men and women.
- *Heart disease.* According to one study, women who took 1 gram of calcium daily experienced a fall in their LDL levels and a corresponding increase in their HDL levels.

Calcium is found in:

- Dairy products
- Salmon and canned salmon, especially in the bones
- Tuna
- Beans
- Soy products
- Sardines and oolichans (very rich sources but also acquired tastes)
- Tofu
- Almonds
- Sesame seeds
- Fortified juices
- Enriched breads
- Collard greens
- Broccoli
- Seaweed
- Chard and kale (What are chard and kale, anyway? Anyone out there ever eaten chard? My son says it may even be kard and chale, so who says eight years on a B.A. was a waste, eh?)

IRON: A BRIDGE TO MORE ENERGY?

You want to think hard about iron, an essential component of hemoglobin, which transports oxygen to your tissues through the bloodstream.

On the one hand, iron deficiency can lead to developmental and be-havioral problems in infants and has been associated with learning and behavior difficulties in young girls. As well, several recent studies have linked low iron levels with excess fatigue in young and middle-aged adults, especially menstruating females.

So why shouldn't everyone take iron supplements? Because (here's that other hand) high stores of iron have been linked to potentially higher risks of heart disease, diabetes, liver disease, and a host of other conditions (this is especially a problem for people who suffer from that disorder known as hemochromatosis, in which too much iron from the diet is absorbed and stored). That's because iron seems to accelerate the production of free radicals and the oxidation of LDL, leading to greater oxidative damage, especially in the heart and blood vessels.

Also, taking iron supplements not only renders meaningless that very important colon cancer screening test, the stool test for occult blood (see chapter 11), by leading to false positive results, it can even hide the anemia that comes on with colon cancer and thus delay diag-nosis. So contrary to the ads that try to convince you that all you need when you have chronic fatigue is a bit more iron, if you are feeling list-less and tired, do not take iron supplements to give you a boost of en-ergy. Instead, find out the reason for your lack of energy, and then, if appropriate, you can take those supplements.

Iron is found in large amounts in and is most easily obtained from:

- Red meat
- Poultry
- Eggs
- Liver
- Legumes
- Walnuts
- Soybeans
- Fish
- Enriched breads and cereals
- Peanut butter
- Tofu
- Seafood

Iron is also available from grains and from fruits such as raisins and apricots, though iron is generally not as well absorbed from such sources.

POTASSIUM: A BANANA A DAY KEEPS THE DOCTOR AWAY

This one is easy to push because potassium is in so many yummy foods. I mean, who doesn't like bananas and strawberries and OJ (besides the LAPD, that is)? And the great thing is that potassium is so good for you.

Several studies have determined that a diet high in potassium helps keep blood pressure down and subsequently leads to a lower risk of stroke. This fact is an especially important consideration for anyone taking diuretics to treat high blood pressure, because many diuretics promote potassium excretion (yes, that means you pee it out). Also, in a study from California, women who ate potassium-rich foods experienced a reduction in normal calcium loss.

You get potassium from:

- Bananas
- Strawberries
- Avocados
- Green, leafy veggies
- Milk
- Nuts
- Tomatoes
- Orange juice
- Spinach
- Melons
- Potatoes
- Meat

SALT (SODIUM): DASH IT ALL

OK, here's another tough one for me. I have trouble telling people to limit their salt intake mainly because several of my basic food groups— olives, pickles, hummus, feta, and smoked meat, but only if you can get it from Schwartz's in Montreal—are loaded with salt. Not only that, a good study in the *British Medical Journal* concluded that it's just so bloody hard (I'm paraphrasing the British here) to lower salt in the diet and it leads to such a small overall drop in blood pressure that it's simply not worth the effort. (To be fair, the DASH [Dietary Approaches to Stop Hypertension] diet study did find that a large group of people could lower their salt intake, but I'm always wary of such studies. Although you can get people to make that kind of change in a study—when you monitor them, when you encourage them, when you take a real interest in what they're doing—it's much harder to get people to make similar changes in the real world where no one cares about them—except for me, of course.)

That said, a diet high in extra salt is clearly not good for many of you, since it can lead to higher blood pressure (and fluid retention) and consequent higher risks of heart attack, heart failure, and stroke. The funny thing about salt, though, is that it clearly doesn't harm many people who use it to excess; lots of people are "immune" to salt's effects. My dad, for example, complained loudly during every meal that my mother had yet again failed to add enough salt—bait she rose to every time, by the way—yet my dad lived into his eighties with absolutely normal blood pressure, though he caused everyone around him to develop high blood pressure. My dad was what the experts call "salt-insensitive" (he was insensitive to a lot of other things, too), one of those lucky people who are able to add oodles of salt to their diet without suffering higher blood pressure as a result.

Other people, however, are not as lucky or as insensitive as my dad, and their blood pressures do rise in response to increasing amounts of sodium in the diet, though the degree of sensitivity to salt can vary quite significantly from the very sensitive to the slightly sensitive. So how do you know if you're salt-sensitive? You don't, and since there is really no easy way to tell how responsive you are to salt intake, the best advice is to simply limit your intake of extra salt (this holds especially true if you've been diagnosed with high blood pressure, since the majority of hypertensives are considered to be salt-sensitive).

Thus, a study of over 17,000 American adults concluded that those who kept their sodium intake down had a much better chance of keeping their blood pressure down than those who didn't limit their sodium intake. Another study found that women who exercised to lower their blood pressures got much better results from the exercise if they also limited their salt intake.

Even more impressively, the aforementioned DASH diet, which emphasizes fruits, veggies, whole grains, poultry, fish, low-fat dairy products, and nuts, has been shown to lower high blood pressure as effectively as the best blood-pressure-lowering drugs, but adults on the DASH diet who also limit their salt intake have even greater decreases in blood pressure than those on the DASH diet alone. In fact, in this study, adults who had a "typical American diet" were also able to lower their blood pressure simply by limiting their salt intake, but I would say that the minute you limit your salt intake, you're no longer eating anything approaching a typical American diet.

But how much salt is too much salt? Well, as always, I don't think it helps to give exact numbers. Let's just leave it at this: most of the salt in your diet comes from canned or packaged or prepared foods (which are ridiculously high in added salt), so avoid buying these whenever possible and try to limit how much extra salt you add to your own food. Most cooks add too much salt to what they prepare, anyway—except for my mother, that is.

One other potential negative effect from a high-salt diet may be on your bones. In one small Australian study, women with a high salt intake also had more bone loss, and the higher the salt intake, the thinner their bones. The researchers speculated that a high salt intake might prevent the absorption of calcium from the diet.

Vitamins: Vitaminute—What's All the Fuss About?
The reason fruits and vegetables are such powerful disease fighters stems in large part from their vitamin content. Studies invariably find that people who have higher levels of vitamins in their bloodstreams also have lower risks of all sorts of nasty things like heart disease, inflammatory conditions, neurodegenerative diseases like Parkinson's disease, dementia, some cancers, and a host of other health problems.

So if higher vitamin levels are so clearly beneficial, why not just skip the fruits and veggies and instead simply dose yourselves with extra (perhaps even massive) doses of every vitamin that might help you prevent disease and live longer? After all, it's lots easier—and probably cheaper—to buy a three-month supply of lycopene pills, say, or a stash of vitamin-rich fish oil capsules than to go out every few days and buy lycopene-rich tomatoes and (yuck!) bony, smelly, scaly fish. (Actually, if you've ever smelled a fish oil capsule, I'm sure you'll stick with the whole fish.)

And that's certainly what lots of people are doing, because the use of supplements is soaring, and health food store aisles are plugged with people buying vitamins and other supplements by the barrel (though I've got to tell you that I avoid health food stores because the people who shop there are always so earnest and so many of them look so sick, and quite frankly, I worry about what I might catch from them).

The problem with depending on supplements alone, though, is that given how little we currently know about the foods we eat and what happens to nutrients in our bodies, it's premature to link most health benefits to a single or even several components of our diet. True, we *can* connect severe health conditions to deficiencies of certain nutrients, such as scurvy, which is due to an extreme deficiency of vitamin C. But very few among us ingest so little vitamin C that we end up with scurvy, and it's much, much harder to link low (but not dramatically low) vitamin C levels to less prominent symptoms than those of scurvy. (Nevertheless, a recent report concerned the diagnosis of scurvy in a university student who had eaten only junk foods while in school; his parents must wonder why they paid the tuition.)

It gets even more difficult to make these connections when you consider how complex fruits and veggies (and grains and beans) are. A tomato, for example, contains hundreds (probably thousands) of nutrients (many that still have not been discovered), and to pick out lycopene, say, as so many have, as the vitamin component of tomatoes that is most essential in helping lower the risk of prostate cancer is simply presumptuous, if not nuts. It's just as sensible to believe, as I do, that the main reason lycopene from tomatoes may help lower the risk of prostate cancer is that in tomatoes, lycopene is surrounded by hundreds of other nutrients—including just the right amounts of vitamin C, potassium, other carotenoids, and so on—and it's that God-made combination, which cannot be mimicked in pill form, that makes tomato-based lycopene so beneficial (and delicious).

◆ ———————————————————————————————— ◆

NUTRIENTS ARE A TEAM SPORT

Let me give you an analogy, guys. You got your immature baby, hockey star Pavel Bure, there. Sure, Pavel can play hockey. He's Russian, after all, or used to be, so he can skate, even if he won't skate into the corners like good, tough Canadian kids, eh, who can't skate but who can sure fight, and who says fighting isn't part of hockey, eh? Anyway, to win a Stanley Cup, you have to want it more than the other guys and you have to play hockey with a team and as a team. And so far, no one has been able to make Pavel the Pampered play as part of a team, so he's no Stanley Cup winner like my guy, Dougie Gilmour. Well, yah, Dougie hasn't won a Cup since 1989, but hey, he's a Canadian kid, eh? Gotta love him.   ·

Nutrients are like that, too. Got it?

◆ ———————————————————————————————— ◆

CAROTENOIDS

There are over 600 known carotenoids (and more are being discovered every year), and their major importance lies in the fact that they are converted in the body to vitamin A. All carotenoids also have antioxidant effects. The carotenoid beta-carotene (along with vitamin E and vitamin C) is perhaps the best known of the antioxidants.

Carotenoids are responsible for the red, orange, and yellow colors of some veggies. They are found in higher amounts in:

- Red and orange veggies: tomatoes, carrots, sweet potatoes
- Dark green, leafy veggies: spinach, broccoli
- Yellow and orange fruits: melons, peaches, apricots

Antioxidants are supposed to be powerful disease fighters, especially perhaps in preventing heart diseases, but in the best studies, beta-carotene supplementation has not been shown to lower rates of heart disease in humans. Even more surprisingly, it has been shown to be potentially harmful. In one famous study, beta-carotene supplementation was linked to higher rates of lung cancer deaths in smokers. Another study recently published in *The Lancet* concluded that not only does beta-carotene supplementation not reduce the risk of heart disease, it might even slightly increase the risk of dying from all causes—including even heart disease.

VITAMIN A

Vitamin A is found in higher amounts in:

- Meat
- Organ meats, especially liver
- Fish and fish oils
- Eggs
- Butter, cream, milk
- Vitamin-fortified foods

Vitamin A helps maintain:

- Healthy vision
- Bones
- Teeth
- Hair
- The linings of the urinary tract, respiratory tract, and other internal organs
- The immune system

Too much vitamin A can lead to:

- Birth defects
- Hair loss
- Joint pain
- Thinner bones
- Liver enlargement
- Menstrual abnormalities

Lycopene

The only reason I'm mentioning the carotenoid lycopene again (which is present in larger amounts in tomatoes and other red fruits and which has been linked to lower risk of heart disease as well as lower risks of prostate and ovarian cancer) is to tell you that it's most easily absorbed from tomatoes that have been cooked, as in tomato sauce, tomato ketchup, and (yes!) tomato salsa. Woo hoo!

B VITAMINS
There are B vitamins and there are B vitamins—meaning I like some, and I tolerate others.

Vitamin B1 (thiamin)
Vitamin B1 helps in the metabolism of carbohydrates and in nerve function. Thiamin is found in higher amounts in:

- Fish
- Nuts
- Spinach
- Enriched cereals and breads
- Legumes
- Poultry
- Whole grains
- Liver
- Beans
- Meat

Vitamin B2 (riboflavin)
Vitamin B2 is also involved in the metabolism of carbohydrates and protein, as well as in the maintenance of mucous membranes, nerve cells, and vision. Riboflavin is found in higher amounts in:

- Milk and dairy products
- Meat
- Chicken
- Fish
- Dark green veggies
- Cruciferous veggies, such as cabbage
- Enriched cereals
- Beans

- Yogurt
- Eggs

Vitamin B3 (niacin)

Niacin is involved in the maintenance of the nervous system, and one intriguing study found that people who ate higher amounts of niacin-rich foods had significantly lower rates of dementia than those who ate less niacin.

Niacin is also important in food metabolism and is a potent cholesterol-lowering agent. One very publicized study found that the combination of niacin and a cholesterol-lowering agent (a statin drug) was much more effective at getting LDL levels down where you want them than either agent acting alone. The problem with using it more widely, though, is that it produces intense flushing (and can worsen gout) and most people find it hard to take.

Niacin is found in:

- Chicken
- Beef
- Eggs
- Tomatoes
- Nuts
- Legumes
- Enriched cereals
- Carrots
- Liver
- Milk
- Fish

Vitamin B6 (pyridoxine)

Vitamin B6 helps maintain nerve function, vision, and metabolic pathways involved in carbohydrate, fats, and protein metabolism. Pyridoxine is a good one because it can help lower homocysteine levels (though it's not as effective at this task as folic acid is). Vitamin B6 is found in:

- Meat
- Carrots

- Seeds
- Nuts
- Legumes
- Fish
- Chicken
- Eggs
- Liver

One word of caution about vitamin B6: unlike its siblings (the water-soluble vitamins), vitamin B6 can build up into toxic levels—leading to, among other things, nerve damage.

Folic acid: The Rodney Dangerfield of vitamins

The more I learn about folic acid, the more I like this B vitamin. Extra doses of folic acid taken daily during pregnancy can significantly reduce the risk of fetal abnormalities such as spina bifida, anencephaly, and cleft palate, as well as defects in the heart and kidney and (according to a recent study) perhaps even Down's syndrome. All women of childbearing years should take extra doses of folic acid every day, since folic acid works best from the moment of conception on, and it may be too late to start taking it the day your pregnancy is diagnosed, because 50 percent of pregnancies are a surprise (only to the mom, of course; 100 percent of pregnancies are a surprise to the dad). Also, women who take folic acid during pregnancy have been found to have a reduced risk of high blood pressure during the pregnancy, and according to a report from the U.K., folic acid can even cut a child's risk of leukemia if the mom takes it when she's pregnant.

But folic acid is also helpful to people besides young women. Folic acid (along with vitamin B12, and perhaps vitamin B6), can dramatically lower homocysteine levels, so anyone who is known to have high homocysteine levels or who is at high risk for this condition should consider taking extra doses of folic acid. In a major review of homocysteine and folic acid in the *British Medical Journal*, researchers looked at over 100 studies that involved folic acid and came to two conclusions:

- The higher your blood level of homocysteine, the higher your risks of heart attack, stroke, and blood clots in the leg—what's known as deep-vein thrombosis, or DVT. DVT is dangerous because if part of that clot breaks off and travels up the bloodstream, it can lead to a stroke or even sudden death. Deaths from Economy Class Syndrome on airplanes, for example, are a direct result of DVT, and not, as many of you might think, airline food. (The last time I flew Lufthansa, three flight attendants tried to talk me out of choosing the fish. I should have listened to them—it nearly killed me.)

- The best way to lower homocysteine levels is to ingest lots of folic acid (and probably vitamins B12 and B6, too). The study in the *British Medical Journal* estimated that reducing homocysteine levels in the general population by a moderate amount through the more widespread use of folic acid could reduce the risk of heart attack by 16 percent, deep-vein thrombosis by 25 percent, and stroke by 25 percent.

Folic acid works in real life, too, not just in theoretical models. In a recent three-country study (China, the U.K., and Australia), researchers determined that giving supplements of folic acid to a group of test subjects improved the health of their blood vessels (what we call endothelial function) and lowered their levels of homocysteine.

Another potential benefit from folic acid may be in lowering the risk of breast cancer. We know that alcohol intake increases the risk of breast cancer in women and that there is really no known safe level of alcohol intake when it comes to breast cancer (see chapter 6). But we also know that a glass or two of wine every day is a good way to lower the risks of heart attack, stroke, and a host of other health problems.

Happily, in a recent study published in the *Journal of the National Cancer Institute*, researchers determined that high intake of folic acid (along with vitamin B6) reduces the risk of breast cancer, especially for those with the added risk of drinking alcohol regularly. In women who regularly consumed at least one glass of alcohol a day, those with the highest levels of folic acid in their blood were 98 percent less likely to develop breast cancer than women with the lowest levels of folic acid. So, ladies, if you're going to imbibe regularly, you might consider taking folic acid supplements.

There is also some evidence that folic acid supplementation may cut the risk of colon cancer. Folic acid is found in higher amounts in:

- Green, leafy veggies
- Fortified cereals and breads
- Whole grains
- Beans
- Peas
- Fruits, especially oranges and melons
- Veggies, especially asparagus, spinach, broccoli, and corn
- Root veggies
- Peanuts, peanut butter
- Fish, especially salmon and tuna
- Poultry
- Beef

But unless you're very determined, it's not easy to get a lot of folic acid in your diet, so (contrary to what I used to argue) I now believe that many of you should seriously consider taking folic acid in the form of supplements.

Before you all rush off to empty pharmacy shelves of folic acid purely on my advice, though, one important caution: there is no study yet that I know of showing taking extra folic acid actually lowers the risk of getting any of the problems we've discussed (with the exception of birth defects). So, for example, no study has yet shown that taking folic acid supplements to lower homocysteine levels has resulted in reducing the actual rate of heart attack and stroke (even though it makes sense), mostly because such studies are still not finished.

There is also at least one other potential problem with folic acid supplementation you should know about: folic acid can mask a deficiency in vitamin B12, and that can lead to problems, especially in the elderly. If you're going to take extra folic acid, make sure you keep your vitamin B12 levels up, as well.

Vitamin B12: B12 and Between

Low levels of vitamin B12 are much more common than you may think. A study from Tufts University concluded that over 50 percent of adults had either "low normal" levels of or a deficiency of vitamin B12, though these conditions are more common in the elderly, because as we age, we no longer absorb some nutrients as well as we used to.

Low levels of B12 are linked to many problems, including:

- Higher rates of dementia
- Anemia
- Severe nerve damage
- Higher levels of homocysteine

So this is another vitamin you may want to consider taking in supplement form (in concert with folic acid), especially if you're at an age when you still remember how long it took Generalissimo Franco of Spain to die. If you have to ask who Franco was, or worse, where Spain is, then congratulations, GenXer, time is on your side and you may want to wait a while before embarking on a course of B12 supplements.

Vitamin B12 is obtained only from animal sources, such as:

- Meat
- Organ meats
- Fish
- Shellfish
- Eggs
- Cheese

Thus, vegetarians, and especially vegans, must take supplemental vitamin B12 if they don't want to get in trouble. And remember, too, that extra folic acid intake can mask a vitamin B12 deficiency.

VITAMIN C

Vitamin C is an antioxidant that plays a role in forming collagen tissue and in helping enzymes do their jobs. This one is a favorite of the food faddists, and studies have implied that high levels of vitamin C might:

- Protect against esophageal cancer, one of the fastest-growing cancers in North America.
- Lower the risk of heart disease.
- Lower the risk of cataracts.

- Help keep blood pressure down.
- Help fight ulcers.
- Boost the immune system (the one most touted by its proponents), since the adrenal glands, so intimately involved in the fight-or-flight response to stress (see chapter 9), are the Fort Knox of vitamin C.

Despite the lack of "objective" data to verify the claims of vitamin C's abilities, there still may be something to them. I load up on vitamin C when I start to feel a cold coming on, and I'm convinced that my colds are less severe and less prolonged than they used to be before I started this regime. In fact, I even recently converted my son to doing the same. Now he also takes vitamin C at the first hint of a cold, and he, too, swears it works (thus also offering a great example of how hypochondriasis and perhaps superstition run in families).

Colds and flus aside (and extra vitamin C clearly doesn't work in everyone trying to fight a cold), I believe you get more than enough vitamin C in a healthy Mediterranean-style diet, and I don't believe you need to take vitamin C supplements to get any of those other proclaimed benefits. You especially don't need to take extra vitamin C (or its pardner, vitamin E) to battle heart disease and stroke. For example, the WAVE (Women's Angiographic Vitamin and Estrogen) trial found that postmenopausal women with pre-existing heart disease who took hormone replacement therapy or vitamins C or E to prevent further deterioration of their hearts got absolutely no benefit from those regimes. Women on the vitamins actually suffered more heart "events" than did women on placebo, though I'm not about to accuse the vitamins of killing anyone. Let's just say it happened, OK, and leave it at that.

As well, the huge British Heart Protection Study found no benefit at all on heart attack risk from vitamin C supplements.

Vitamin C is found in:

- Oranges and other citrus fruits
- Strawberries
- Peppers, especially red peppers
- Tomatoes
- Potatoes

- Broccoli
- Mangoes and papayas
- Cruciferous vegetables, such as cabbage
- Fish

One word of caution: in very high doses, vitamin C may cause diarrhea and (the jury is still out on this) increase the risk of kidney stones in those people already at high risk for them.

If you do decide to take supplements of vitamin C, please don't believe those people who say that it makes a difference if you take specific forms of the vitamin, such as Ester C. Hey, if we can't even prove that vitamin C makes any difference at all, how in the world can we show that a specific form is better than another? And why is it, I wonder, that none of those vitamin-savvy people ever push the cheapest alternative.

VITAMIN D: NOT ENOUGH HOME-GROWN

Here's another favorite of mine, and along with folic acid and vitamin B12, one I would urge many of you to take in supplement form.

Vitamin D is essential in the absorption of calcium, and hence in the health of bones and teeth, but it also acts like a hormone and plays a key role in cellular health, as well as in maintaining healthy organs and muscles and a healthy brain. Vitamin D is unique among vitamins because our bodies can make it, through exposure to the sun, which helps turn a precursory and inactive form of vitamin D found in our skin into an active form that circulates in our bloodstream to our tissues. All you need to make enough vitamin D is about 10 minutes a day of sun exposure, but most of us, especially those living in more northern areas generally don't get enough sun exposure year-round to make enough of our own home-grown vitamin D. In one study of patients admitted to a Boston-area hospital, nearly 60 percent were deemed to be deficient in vitamin D, including the young.

Given that we might all benefit from higher levels of vitamin D than even the authorities currently recommend, that means a hell of a lot of us are probably deficient in vitamin D—all except my friend Jack, who shouts "Milk!" at waitresses who ask him what beverage he would like. Jack probably has enough vitamin D in him to light up Butte, Montana.

Anyway, most of us may be in need of more vitamin D, and to that end the American Academy of Pediatrics has very recently recommended that even infants, especially those who are breast-fed (breast milk contains little vitamin D), should get vitamin D supplements.

And this may be one hell of a useful vitamin, folks:

- In one study, women over the age of 65 who took vitamin D supplements were able to cut their risk of dying from a heart attack by 33 percent compared with a group of women who didn't take supplements.
- A German study found that women who took vitamin D supplements along with their calcium supplements were able to lower their blood pressures and heart rates better than those who took only calcium supplements.
- Vitamin D has been linked to a lower risk of certain cancers, including colon cancer, prostate cancer, and perhaps breast cancer, too. Breast cancer rates, for example, are higher in the dreary, cloudy, short-day U.S. Northeast than they are in the much sunnier Southwest, and some researchers think that vitamin D may be part of the reason (others believe it may be due to melatonin imbalance); women in the Southwest obviously get to make lots more of it than do women in the Northeast.
- In a recent study, vitamin D supplements increased calcium absorption by a whopping 65 percent.

On the other hand, too much vitamin D can lead to:

- Kidney failure
- Depression
- Liver failure

And, in theory, very high doses of vitamin D can leach calcium out of bone.

Vitamin D is found in:

- Fortified dairy products such as milk
- Eggs

- Oily fish
- Vegetable oils
- Liver

VITAMIN E: DOES IT OR DOESN'T IT?

No matter how ineffective studies show vitamin E to be and no matter how many studies fail to establish that it prevents illness, there are still loads and loads of people out there who fervently believe that if you just give it the proper chance, vitamin E is bound to show you that it really does work. So like a typical, wussy, fence-sitting Canadian, I'm going to give you both sides of this story and let you decide for yourself.

Let me first lay out the anti-vitamin E side, and I warn you, it's quite a roster:

- In a study published in the journal *Circulation*, 11,000 men and women who had recently suffered a heart attack were divided into three groups. One group got "usual care" (meaning watchful waiting and the latest medications), the second group got vitamin E, and the third group got only fish oil capsules (the researchers probably had it in for that last group). To quote the authors: "The vitamin E did nothing to alter the risk of heart disease."
- In the previously mentioned WAVE study, women who received vitamin E actually had more subsequent heart attacks than did women who only got placebo, though no one is willing to say that the vitamin E was responsible for this surprising result. It's much more likely, everyone hems and haws, that this unexpected finding was purely a result of chance.
- In the HOPE (Heart Outcomes Prevention Evaluation) study, the arm of the study dedicated to the use of vitamin E found, I'm sure you've guessed, absolutely no benefit in preventing heart problems from taking vitamin E.
- In the British Heart Protection Study, in which researchers showed that people with normal cholesterol levels who have certain other risk factors for cardiac problems would still benefit enormously from taking cholesterol-lowering drugs, the researchers also found absolutely no benefit from taking vitamin E.
- Finally, in the Honolulu-Asia Aging Study, men who took vitamin E

and vitamin C supplements suffered no less dementia than did men who eschewed vitamin intervention (chewers and eschewers were essentially equal, in other words).

So what do the see-no-evil UN inspectors say to that mountain of evidence? You guessed: just give it another chance, boys, because "the next time, it will comply." And they point to small bits of evidence, such as these, to push their opinion:

- Some studies have concluded that daily use of vitamin E reduces heart disease and slows progression of already-existing heart disease.
- The Baltimore Longitudinal Study of Aging found a significant reduction in Alzheimer's disease in those with a higher blood level of vitamin E.
- The Nurses' Health Study and the Health Professionals Follow-Up Study found a reduced risk of Parkinson's disease with higher intake of vitamin E.
- In some studies, people with higher blood levels of vitamin E have scored higher in tests of cognition than those with lower vitamin E levels.
- Better lung function has been found with higher levels of vitamin E.
- Higher levels of vitamin E have been linked with lower levels of prostate cancer.

So there you have it, folks. On this one, I'm afraid, you pays yer money and you takes yer chances. And if you decide vitamin E is for you, you do pays yer money, because it's impossible to get the higher doses commonly recommended from diet alone, so you have to buy some type of vitamin E supplement.

Natural sources of vitamin E include:

- Vegetable oils and seed oils (soybean, wheat germ, corn, cottonseed, sunflower)
- Avocados
- Eggs
- Liver

- Whole grains
- Peanut butter
- Nuts
- Beans
- Brown rice
- Wheat germ

And though these are probably very rare occurrences, too much vitamin E can theoretically lead to:

- Clotting problems
- Deficiencies of other vitamins

VITAMIN K

This vitamin is primarily involved in blood-clotting and is also important to bone health. Vitamin K is made in your gastrointestinal tract by bacteria that reside there and manufacture it from:

- Dark green, leafy veggies
- Oils
- Soybeans
- Molasses (who eats molasses?)
- Eggs
- Some legumes
- Cruciferous veggies
- Milk

Too much vitamin K can lead to clotting problems.

5

Eating for
Weight Control

*The Dr. Art Hister Surefire Way to Lose 20
Pounds in 10 Days While Eating All You Can
Eat (and Other Myths)*

I don't diet. I just don't eat as much as I'd like to.
LINDA EVANGELISTA

L ET ME NOW turn to the real reason most of you
have read this far: you want to know if I have
a painless and surefire way to help you lose
lots of weight quickly, preferably within several hours, though you
might be willing to wait a couple of weeks if I can promise that my diet
plan is absolutely bound to help you keep those pounds off.

Well, I'm afraid I can't promise you that kind of quick result. I can,
however, promise you that if you are willing to be patient, and if you
are willing to stick with my suggestions, you will eventually lose
significant amounts of weight (if that's your goal), and even more important, you will have an excellent chance of keeping those pounds off.
First, though, let me ask you this poser: besides your spouse's constantly
telling you that you need to lose some weight, how do you know that
you really are overweight?

So How Fat Are You?

The most common method of figuring out where you stand weight-wise is to calculate your BMI, which stands for body mass index. The BMI is calculated by multiplying your weight in kilograms by 10,000 and dividing that number by your height in centimeters squared.

But for those of you who may need help with the maths on this one, or want to convert from pounds and inches, I am including a BMI table. There you will discover that a BMI of 25 is the dividing line between desired weight and weighing too much. Thus, if your BMI is under 25, you're OK; if it's over 25, you're overweight; if your BMI is over 30, you're considered obese; and if your BMI is over 40 you're extrememly obese (see following page for BMI chart).

Sounds simple enough, but as usual it's not, because there are many problems with using BMI as the sole measure for deciding whether your weight is ideal or not. Most important—and this will scare you, I assure you—a couple of large studies, including the Nurses' Health Study and the Health Professionals Study, found that rates of heart disease, high blood pressure, colon cancer, gallstones, and diabetes actually start to climb not from a BMI of 25 but from a BMI in the range of 22. Ouch!

Another problem with BMI as the sole marker of ideal weight is that if you were slimmer as a young adult—with, say, a BMI of 20 (and yes, there are people like that, such as my obnoxious wife, who have always been *thin*)—and if you gain 20 or 30 pounds later in life, you still retain a "normal" BMI level (somewhere around 24 to 25), yet you would still have gained enough weight to negatively affect your health. Several studies, including the Framingham Study, indicate that any weight gain at all after young adulthood affects health adversely.

If like me, however, you were once fat and you have managed to build up some muscle to replace some of your old fat tissue, your BMI won't come down as much as it would have had you simply set out to lose weight, since muscle tissue weighs more than fat tissue—though you would still have become much healthier. Also, BMI doesn't account at all for *where* you store your fat, and as you no doubt remember from chapter 1, abdominal fat is way worse for you than fat stored elsewhere. Someone with a BMI of 26, say, whose fat stores

BODY MASS INDEX TABLE

BMI	Normal						Overweight					Obese										Extreme Obesity			
	19	20	21	22	23	24	25	26	27	28	29	30	31	32	33	34	35	36	37	38	39	40	41	42	43
HEIGHT												BODY WEIGHT (pounds)													
58"	91	96	100	105	110	115	119	124	129	134	138	143	148	153	158	162	167	172	177	181	186	191	196	201	205
59"	94	99	104	109	114	119	124	128	133	138	143	148	153	158	163	168	173	178	183	188	193	198	203	208	212
60"	97	102	107	112	118	123	128	133	138	143	148	153	158	163	168	174	179	184	189	194	199	204	209	215	220
61"	100	106	111	116	122	127	132	137	143	148	153	158	164	169	174	180	185	190	195	201	206	211	217	222	227
62"	104	109	115	120	126	131	136	142	147	153	158	164	169	175	180	186	191	196	202	207	213	218	224	229	235
63"	107	113	118	124	130	135	141	146	152	158	163	169	175	180	186	191	197	203	208	214	220	225	231	237	242
64"	110	116	122	128	134	140	145	151	157	163	169	174	180	186	192	197	204	209	215	221	227	232	238	244	250
65"	114	120	126	132	138	144	150	156	162	168	174	180	186	192	198	204	210	216	222	228	234	240	246	252	258
66"	118	124	130	136	142	148	155	161	167	173	179	186	192	198	204	210	216	223	229	235	241	247	253	260	266
67"	121	127	134	140	146	153	159	166	172	178	185	191	198	204	211	217	223	230	236	242	249	255	261	268	274
68"	125	131	138	144	151	158	164	171	177	184	190	197	203	210	216	223	230	236	243	249	256	262	269	276	282
69"	128	135	142	149	155	162	169	176	182	189	196	203	209	216	223	230	236	243	250	257	263	270	277	284	291
70"	132	139	146	153	160	167	174	181	188	195	202	209	216	222	229	236	243	250	257	264	271	278	285	292	299
71"	136	143	150	157	165	172	179	186	193	200	208	215	222	229	236	243	250	257	265	272	279	286	293	301	308
72"	140	147	154	162	169	177	184	191	199	206	213	221	228	235	242	250	258	265	272	279	287	294	302	309	316
73"	144	151	159	166	174	182	189	197	204	212	219	227	235	242	250	257	265	272	280	288	295	302	310	318	325
74"	148	155	163	171	179	186	194	202	210	218	225	233	241	249	256	264	272	280	287	295	303	311	319	326	334
75"	152	160	168	176	184	192	200	208	216	224	232	240	248	256	264	272	279	287	295	303	311	319	327	335	343
76"	156	164	172	180	189	197	205	213	221	230	238	246	254	263	271	279	287	295	304	312	320	328	336	344	353

Source: Adapted from Clinical Guidelines on the Identification, Evaluation, and Treatment of Overweight and Obesity in Adults: The Evidence Report

are mainly around the middle, is at considerably more risk of problems than someone with a similar BMI who keeps her fat mainly on her hips and butt.

But hey, imperfect though it is, BMI is still a convenient and acceptably accurate approximation of the relative health risks you face from your fat stores. It's used in most studies about weight and its attendant health risks.

Why Is It So Bad to Be Obese?
Obesity has been linked to higher risks of many significant health problems:

- Overall mortality. Obesity has been estimated to account for between 7 percent and 30 percent of all deaths in developed countries. In the U.S., according to Dr. Julie Gerberding, director of the Centers for Disease Control and Prevention, obesity has now nearly caught up to tobacco as the leading preventable cause of death.
- Heart disease, including heart attacks, heart failure, sudden death, and other problems. In the Framingham Study, the Nurses' Health Study, and the Cancer Prevention Study, obesity was an independent risk factor for heart disease mortality, meaning that it's a risk factor even after you account for high cholesterol, high blood pressure, and so on.
- High blood pressure. Your risk of high blood pressure is seven times as great if you're obese as if you're not, and dropping even a few pounds can lead to a significant drop in blood pressure.
- Strokes. One study estimates that each unit increase in BMI is associated with a 6 percent increased risk of stroke; another study estimates that being overweight by as little as 2.7 kilograms (6 pounds) is enough to raise the risk of stroke.
- Blood clots. Not only are overweight adults more likely to end up with blood clots, but studies also show that preventive measures such as wearing leg-compression stockings will not work for them nearly as well as they work for people of normal weight.
- All sorts of cancers: prostate (obese men have double the risk of getting hit in the end), uterine, gallbladder, pancreatic, kidney, colon, and breast (women who are slim not only have a lower risk of

getting breast cancer than more robust women but also have a higher rate of surviving breast cancer).

- Insulin resistance and diabetes. Fifty-seven percent of all diabetes cases have been attributed to obesity, and your risk of diabetes is six times as high if you're obese. Also, and this is really sad, Type 2 diabetes cases are exploding among our youth. Then there's the metabolic syndrome, which is a very hot issue these days: nearly a quarter of Americans are currently said to have the metabolic syndrome, and the rate is rising rapidly with the spreading waistlines that plague the U.S. population.

◆ ————————————————————————— ◆

WHAT IS THE METABOLIC SYNDROME?

The metabolic syndrome is a collection of health problems that includes:

- Insulin resistance
- Cholesterol abnormalities, especially low HDL and high triglycerides (known officially as dyslipidemia)
- High blood pressure
- High blood sugar
- The physical feature of abdominal obesity

These features are so linked that according to the U.S. Prevention Services Task Force, anyone who has high blood pressure or high cholesterol should be screened for diabetes. Because none of these problems produce obvious signs of symptoms (aside from the clear increase in girth), most people with the metabolic syndrome don't know they have it.

The metabolic syndrome raises your subsequent health risks—heart attack, stroke, even early memory loss (some of you might want to take notes here before you forget this)—especially, perhaps, if you're a woman.

◆ ————————————————————————— ◆

Other health problems associated with obesity include:

- GERD.
- Gallbladder disease.
- Chronic inflammation. Obese men and women have significantly higher levels of CRP—you remember CRP, I'm sure, from chapter 1—than those who are of normal weight.
- Osteoarthritis. Obese teenage girls are much more likely to eventually require hip replacement than are girls of normal weight.
- Sleep apnea—a condition in which breathing is obstructed during sleep, leading to a temporary cessation of breathing and consequent gasps of fear from the sleeping partner (see chapter 8).
- Mental health problems. In kids, a recent eight-year study found a strong link between obesity and "psychiatric" conditions such as behavior problems and depression. Another study found—very sadly—that severely obese kids rate their quality of life to be as low as that of kids who are on chemotherapy. In adults, average weights have gone up so much that there may no longer be as much of a stigma associated with being overweight as there was once, but obese people are still more likely to suffer from depression and other psychiatric conditions. And weight clearly plays an important role in self-image; 24 percent of women and 17 percent of men responded in a *Psychology Today* survey that they would give up three years of their lives to be thinner. In kids, a survey from Pennsylvania State University found a negative self-image in overweight girls as young as five years old.
- Poor lung function.
- Age-related macular degeneration and cataracts.
- Urinary incontinence if you're female.
- Lower IQs. A recent study found that men with a BMI over 30 performed worse on IQ tests than men with a normal BMI. A Canadian study found that overweight people complain of poorer cognitive functioning. (How can you tell if a Canadian is becoming demented? Take your choice: he actually stands for something; he doesn't ask the government for handouts; he stops being polite.)
- Difficulty getting pregnant, even with in vitro fertilization.

- In women, increased risk of having babies with birth defects such as spina bifida and heart abnormalities.
- Being killed or seriously injured in motor vehicle accidents.
- Suffering disability in daily living.

Being overweight also costs you plenty—and in Canada, it costs me, too. One American study found that obese women between the ages of 57 and 68 had net worths of about $135,000 less than their nonobese sisters. But there are also huge direct costs from being obese. One study recently estimated that obesity exacts higher health care costs than either smoking or drinking alcohol. In another study, researchers followed employees of a large American company and concluded that the average extra health costs for an obese individual totaled roughly $1,500 a year. When you think about how quickly the rates of obesity have been escalating, "Ohmigawd" is all I can say about how high health care costs will soon rise.

Perhaps the worst effect of obesity is that fat parents have fat kids, and to put it bluntly, folks, our kids are ballooning. According to one estimate, in Canada there are now more fat kids as a proportion of the total kid population than the corresponding proportion of fat adults in the adult population. More than a third of Canadian kids between the ages of two and 11 are now overweight (and half of these are obese), while a staggering 25 percent of Canadian kids aged two to three are now considered obese. In the U.S. the number of overweight kids has tripled since 1980, and obesity has really skyrocketed among black and Mexican-American children. This spreading trend has no end in sight, and has led one British expert to claim that if kids in the developed world continue to get fatter at current rates, obesity is going to reverse the gains in longevity that have been built up over the past century—that is, our kids will die at younger ages than we are likely to.

Sadly, the younger you are when you're overweight, the worse it is for you. According to the Bogalusa Heart Study, overweight adolescents are much more likely than adolescents of normal weight to end up as young adults with abnormal cholesterol levels and are eight times as likely to end up with high blood pressure, which will eventually lead to far higher rates of heart attacks, strokes, and dementia. These complications are also likely to occur at a much younger age in fat kids than in normal-weight kids.

According to a British study that tracked over 10,000 students for more than 40 years, overweight adolescents are also at increased risk of dying from cancer (prostate cancer in the guys, breast cancer in the fems) later in life compared with normal-weight kids.

Bottom line, though, is this: according to statistics, your wishes, and what we know about the health consequences of being overweight, most of you—and your kids—should probably lose some weight. The question is how best to do it.

How Can You Lose Weight?

COUNSELING

Start with a doctor who's willing to help you. Make sure, however, that the doctor you choose is slim herself. Studies show that weight loss is more easily achieved with the help and advice of a caring health professional, but they also show that the best advice comes from doctors who practice what they preach. You have a much greater chance of losing weight when you're under the guidance of a doctor of either sex who looks like Hilary Swank than of one who looks like Zero Mostel.

DRUGS

Weight-loss drugs do work somewhat. A recent major review of studies involving anti-obesity drugs concluded that they help some people, though overall they lead to a maximum long-term weight loss of about 5 percent of body weight, a level of weight loss, I submit, that should be attainable for most people without the aid of medications.

The review also determined that all the studies done with anti-obesity drugs had high attrition rates, meaning that people just don't like being on the drugs. It's also important to remember that weight-loss drugs don't have the best track record as far as safety is concerned, so even though the ones on the market now are considered to be safe, one small part of my brain still keeps repeating, "Fen-Phen, Fen-Phen, Fen-Phen."

If you want to lose weight and keep it off, seems to me that you should not seek a quick chemical cure but instead learn to readjust your eating habits. You're going to have to do that sooner or later, anyway.

CALORIE RESTRICTION

So, let's move along to the only thing we do know for sure about losing weight: *the less you eat, the less you will weigh.* Guaranteed. Every single person in history who has been forced to endure a prolonged famine has subsequently become emaciated as a result of the calorie restriction. Period. No exceptions.

If you restrict your calorie intake enough, you will lose weight, and curiously, significant calorie restriction may also lead to other positive health consequences. At least it does in animals. Specifically, in some species, cutting calories by 30 to 40 percent has been shown to postpone many of the changes associated with "normal aging" and to increase longevity by an amazing 30 percent.

In a study from the University of Wisconsin, researchers concluded that in mice calorie restriction retards the aging process of the heart by impeding genes involved in changes associated with aging, even when the reduced calorie intake doesn't start until middle age. Higher up the evolutionary ladder we come to dogs (though I sincerely doubt that my malamute, Big Louie, could beat an advanced mouse in an IQ showdown—he can't follow a straight path, never mind navigate a maze). Dogs fed a calorie-restricted diet lived up to two years longer, the equivalent of 14 human years, and had fewer degenerative conditions (such as arthritis) associated with aging. A study that is still under way is finding that monkeys also live longer when they eat less.

Why might calorie restriction lead to longer life and perhaps better health, too? Well, in the lab, scientists have discovered that calorie restriction leads to much lower levels of free radicals, better hormone levels, less cell death, better muscle and nerve function, and better blood chemistry (lipid levels, blood glucose, and so on).

In humans, there are no studies similar to those done on rodents and dogs (there is, of course, a wee ethical problem in restricting people's access to eating as much as they want), yet we may eventually have some empirical evidence whether things work the same in humans; a few brave but idiotic souls claim to be eating 30 to 40 percent fewer calories than average in an attempt to live longer. (The easy joke is that they may not actually live any longer, but they will surely feel as if they had. I also often wonder if these folks ever get depressed and ask themselves, "But what if I'm wrong?") The answer will become available either 10, 20, 30, 40, 50, or 60 years from now.

Although there is no direct proof that calorie restriction extends life in humans, there is lots of evidence that calorie restriction promotes better health. One small study in severely overweight people found that a very low calorie diet led to "immediate improvement" (less than one month) in several markers of heart health, causing the lead author to exclaim, "Every piece of excess food you eat is an insult to the body." (If that excess food is chocolate, then I say, "Insult me, insult me. I can handle it.") The bad news, though, is that as soon as these folks abandoned their diets, those markers started shooting up, and some markers rose to even higher levels than before the diet had started.

In Biosphere 2, a group of morons—excuse me, a group of researchers—was willingly locked away in a big dome for two years. As part of the researchers' confinement, they started to eat less. As their calories dropped, their blood markers for aging and other health parameters improved—specifically, their weights, blood pressures, blood sugar levels, insulin levels, and cholesterol levels dropped. In the Baltimore Longitudinal Study on Aging published in the journal *Science*, researchers found that men who lived the longest tended to have levels of biological markers—low basal body temperature, low insulin levels, and low levels of certain hormones—that are found in animals that live longer as a result of calorie restriction (though none of the men in this study were consciously restricting calorie intake in an attempt to live longer). So eating far less may be good for you, but given that most of us prefer to eat 30 percent *more* than we're supposed to, I doubt that extreme calorie restriction will become the next great fad to rival, say, playing hackysack or watching *American Idol*.

FAT RESTRICTION

As we've seen, severely reducing total calorie intake does lead to weight loss, but most people don't seem to have the capacity to restrict calorie intake for a long time. This is why a huge diet industry has erupted that has as its basic tenet a "biochemical" explanation for how to limit only specific food groups to lose weight—thus, in theory, allowing dieters to eat as much as they'd like. The best known of these diets is the fat-restriction diet, whose practitioners advise that you can achieve significant weight loss simply by restricting fats. After all, fat provides more than twice as many calories per gram as carbohydrates (9 versus 4). Trouble is, restricting fats simply doesn't work.

A mountain of data points to the same conclusion: although low-fat diets have been in vogue for years and some low-fat dieters have indeed lost weight for a while (and a few have managed to lose many kilograms and keep most of them off, too), the large majority of low-fat dieters have put those lost kilos on again over time. Not only that, for poorly understood reasons, most low-fat-diet followers have gone on to weigh even more than they did before they started dieting.

A detailed two-decade survey of Minnesota residents found that although their average fat consumption fell steadily during those 20 years, obesity levels (and average cholesterol levels) in that population climbed just as steadily over that time. In Europe, a report from Datamonitor showed that fewer than 1 in 50 European dieters "achieve permanent weight loss" on diets, despite statistics telling us that Europeans spend the "equivalent of the economic output of Morocco" every year on low-fat-diet products. The bottom line? We are eating less fat in North America (it's down from 40 percent of the diet two decades ago to 34 or 35 percent of the diet now), but we weigh more than ever.

Restricting fat intake somewhat, then, does not seem to be the answer if you're trying to lose weight, especially not when it's married to the outrageous advice to replace those fats with as many carbohydrates as you would like to eat. I mean, who in the world besides late-20th-century Boobus Americanus could have convinced himself that he could lose weight on a diet of unlimited white bread, pasta, potato dishes, starches, sweets, and so on, as long as those products were "low-fat"?

So, we're not doing well on our own by restricting fats somewhat. But what about some of those very famous diets that so many people follow? Do they give you a better shot at losing weight?

THE DEAN ORNISH DIET

The Dean Ornish diet is a very low-fat/high-carb diet in which the carbohydrates are all high-fiber foods. There is good evidence that the Dean Ornish diet does work: it not only inevitably leads to weight loss if you stick with it but also seems to produce significant long-term improvements in cholesterol levels and insulin resistance (and perhaps to the risks of certain cancers, too). The most likely reason the Dean Ornish diet is so successful in helping people who stick to it lose weight, though, is that they end up ingesting fewer calories.

This diet is hard to stick with, however. I know of many people who have done the Dean Ornish diet—for a while. Eventually, they all seem to give up—they just want more fats in their diet. In fact, they crave fats, and so they go off the diet and generally regain their weight. That said, if you want to lose weight and get mellow at the same time, Dean Ornish's diet and health plan (which also has a strong emphasis on stress reduction, exercise, and total wellness) is a good way to go.

And by the way, even Dean Ornish himself admits to eating a "little bit" of chocolate every day.

THE DR. ATKINS DIET

Then there's a guy who not only didn't restrict fat intake in his diet but encouraged you to eat as much fat as you wanted—very weird advice to those of us trained on the mantra that fat is ugly. (It seems strange to put all this in the past; I miss Dr. Atkins, because he stirred things up, and we need more people to do that in this complacent and staid medical business.) The Atkins diet (high, high, high protein; high, high, high fat; and low, low, low carbohydrates) does lead to weight loss. I've seen many friends and patients lose vast quantities of corporeal real estate in relatively short periods of time on the Atkins diet.

Although most of the studies involving Atkins dieters have been small and short-term, they are also pretty consistent in their conclusions: this diet works. In one important study (funded by the Robert Atkins Foundation), originally skeptical Duke University researchers enrolled 120 people in a head-to-head battle between the Atkins diet and the standard Duke U high-carb, low-fat diet, and the Atkins diet won a clear victory.

After six months, Atkinsonians lost an average of 14 kilograms (31 pounds), compared with 9 kilograms (20 pounds) for the high-carbers. But the really eye-opening margins of victory were seen in blood chemistry results: the Atkins people had an 11 percent rise in HDL and a 49 percent drop in triglycerides, while the low-fatties had only a 1 percent rise in HDL and a 22 percent drop in triglyceride levels (and bear in mind that several studies have shown that in lowering the risk of heart disease, it may be most important to raise HDL).

Game to Dr. Atkins.

In two recent studies published in the *New England Journal of Medicine* comparing the Atkins diet to traditional low-fat diets, the Atkins diet was the clear winner—better weight loss, better lipid blood levels—at both six months and a year.

Game, set, and match to Dr. Atkins.

But now for the inevitable provisos.

First, despite the protestations of its acolytes that biochemistry makes the Atkins diet so effective (a high-animal-protein diet, for example, increases blood levels of leucine, which in turn helps maintain muscle mass and reduce body fat), the reality is that there is probably nothing magical in the Atkins formula and the main reason for its success is not biochemistry but plain old calorie reduction. For anyone with even a modest sense of taste, the Atkins diet is boring beyond belief (as a method writer, I tried Atkins once, but I lasted only two days because protein and fat are just so damn *borrrrring* when you can't balance them with lots of different veggies, spuds, grains, etc.). So I am certain that most Atkins dieters probably restrict their calorie intake because you can only eat so much beef before barfing, and that's really why they lose weight. In fact, that's been the conclusion of every one of those studies I cited earlier—namely, that low-carb diets owe their success mainly to the consequent calorie restriction that happens on such diets.

Second, I have yet to meet anyone—anyone—who has kept the weight they lost on Atkins off over the long term. My dozens of acquaintances who lost weight on Atkins all eventually went off the diet and quickly regained every pound they'd lost. Many of them even added on a lot of extra weight for good measure. Now I know that the Atkins people will vehemently protest that those poor results are not the fault of the diet but rather the fault of people who didn't stick to something that was working, but hey, guys, if very few people manage to stick to a diet, don't you think it's really the fault of the diet and not the dieter?

Third, there is no evidence that the Atkins diet is safe over the long term (a couple of studies have suggested that the Atkins diet may lead to a higher risk of bone loss and kidney stones, as well as a higher risk of dehydration with excess exercise, but those findings need to be verified in larger studies). True, people have been on Atkins (more accurately, they've been on it and off it) for over 30 years, but no one knows what's happened to these folks. Have they flourished? Are there a large number of supermodels among them? Have they won a disproportionate number of Nobel prizes? Have some of them defected to North Korea? Most worryingly, what has happened to their cardiovascular systems from years of ingesting animal fat and protein? No one knows, and that's not very reassuring.

So until there are more data, I would avoid this diet (except if you really, really need it for short-term bursts to beef up your belief in your ability to lose weight).

But if, like my kids, you choose to completely ignore my advice, and you do the Atkins diet, anyway, as I'm sure many of you will, then bear this in mind: a recent study found that those low-carb energy bars that everyone uses on these diets for snacks and instant energy hits don't actually keep insulin levels down. Contrary to what the manufacturers of these bars would have you believe, the low-carb, high-protein bars that were tested in this study led to a pretty good spike in insulin levels, and the best food in keeping insulin levels down in this limited study was—are you ready?—chicken. So even as we speak, I'm trying to get a group of investors to come up with a quick-energy chicken bar. Another of my great can't-lose schemes, eh?

THE ZONE DIET
The Zone diet operates on the 40-30-30 plan (40 percent carbohydrates, 30 percent protein, 30 percent fat), which is how you get insulin and something else called eicosanoids (these play an important role in helping you deal with inflammation) into the right "zone," which in turn will help you lose weight and, even more important, regain your health. Like the aforementioned weight-loss diets, the Zone diet also seems to be quite effective in the short term. The Zone diet (which, by the way, is classified as a high-protein diet by the American Heart Association) also focuses on fruits and veggies (and other low-glycemic-index foods—see chapter 3) as the main source of carbohydrates, which is mostly a good thing, and on eating more often during the day, which is also a good thing, as long as you snack on healthy foods.

The problem is that people on this diet tend to become obsessed with food proportions, and to me, that's unhealthy, unrealistic, and unsustainable in the long run. Most people are just not able to stick to a plan if they have to apportion protein or calculate carbs, and they will very likely abandon the effort out of sheer frustration. Indeed, the cumbersome calculations are such a burden that software is available to help you figure out what to eat, and if you need a calculator or computer to stick with your diet, better get another diet, folks.

Finally, most experts agree that as with the Atkins diet, most people lose weight on this diet primarily because they consume fewer calories.

What Really Works?

The weight of evidence clearly shows that these very popular diets have not made very many of us any slimmer. In fact, we've just continued to grow and grow and grow.

So is the big, fat bottom line that we are doomed to get bigger by the year, since nothing can help us lose weight and keep it off? No, no, and no. You can lose weight and keep it off, and I say that because lots of people have done it. You see, lurking among us is an anonymous army of millions of what are called "successful losers" ("successful losers" is not an oxymoron when it applies to weight, accents, and occasionally spouses). And studies tell us that successful losers have some tactics in common that help them lose weight and keep those pounds off— tactics that we can all develop, I think.

A survey of 32,000 dieters by *Consumer Reports* found that the great majority of people who kept weight off for more than a year:

- Considered exercise the key to their weight loss.
- Didn't use any special diet or diet gimmick.

Not too complicated, eh? Even more impressive, an American study of 3,000 successful losers who had dumped an average of 30 kilograms (66 pounds) and kept them off for an average of five and a half years found that most of them:

- Did lots of exercise, in the range of one hour a day nearly every day of the week.

- Never skipped meals.
- Tended to eat healthy and hearty breakfasts. (See? I told you break-fast was important.)
- Obsessively watched how much they ate, especially portion sizes, and (contrary to what many weight-loss experts advise) they also watched their weight obsessively, often weighing themselves several times a day. (I suppose that as soon as they noticed a gain they were unhappy with, they compensated by exercising more and perhaps by eating less, too.)
- Claimed to follow a low-fat, high-carb diet, but I believe this diet was incidental to their success—I think these folks would have been equally successful on any diet.

I know this regimen works, because it is pretty much what I have done. Thus, the secret to my successful losing is not, as my wife would have it, that I am clearly good at losing, but rather because I do most of the things I just told you about. I've lost nearly 18 kilograms (40 pounds)—well, 17.1 kilos (37.8 pounds) as of my last weigh-in, about 19.5 minutes ago—which I've managed to keep off for over three years (actually, 38.5 months), because I do lots of exercise, I adhere to a relatively modest Mediterranean diet, I never skip meals (my first-thing-in-the-morning muffin with its subsequent prompt visit to the can is the stuff of legend around our house, if "legend" is the right word to use for something that makes everyone laugh at me), and I watch my weight very closely. When I gain a few pounds (after a trip, for example), I compensate with what my sons call "Dad's punishment"—extra exercise. And it works!

Exercise has been the key to my keeping weight off, but next in line has definitely been my conversion to the Mediterranean-style diet, in large part because it's such a rich diet in which I can eat so many varied foods—*in moderation*. That keeps me very happy, not to mention that it allows me to eat in a much more sensible way without (horrors!) that daunting—and ultimately defeating—task of calorie counting.

Two last things: First, if you set out to lose weight, please be patient. Losing weight won't—and shouldn't—happen overnight. Like the tortoise, the winners at being the best losers are also often the slowest losers. It took me over a year to lose the weight I lost, but I've kept it all off in large part because I retrained myself to eat right, and that takes time.

Second, if you are going to diet to lose weight, for heaven's sake, be realistic about what you can achieve. One study presented at a recent meeting of the North American Association for the Study of Obesity concluded that even when they're counseled about what goals to aim for, patients still set unrealistic and unachievable goals on diet plans, thus setting themselves up for disappointment and future rebound weight gain. Another study found that women often diet in order to change their body shape, which is, again, generally not a realistic goal.

So you are never going to be as thin as Kate Hudson or even her mom, Vancouver resident Goldie Hawn, no matter how long and how hard you diet, nor should you aim to be. Just a little less of you is probably good enough for most of you.

THE 5 PERCENT RULE

Although there are no formulas, in general, losing 5 percent of body weight is pretty good and attainable; losing 10 percent is great but less attainable (though that is the goal most people should probably shoot for), and only a few ever get beyond 10 percent and keep it off.

CHAPTER

6

Alcohol

Vive La Compagnie!

The first draught serveth for health, the second for
pleasure, the third for shame, the fourth for madness.
SIR WALTER RALEIGH

When I read about the evils of drinking,
I gave up reading.
HENNY YOUNGMAN

K EEPING WITH MY COMMITMENT to stay completely honest in this book, I have to tell you
that I'm writing this while sitting on the
beach in Mexico, sipping a daiquiri, and wondering about my stock
portfolio. (My broker likes to joke that my portfolio has plunged more
than Halle Berry's décolletage, though I wonder if he'll still be making
jokes when he's out on parole and he has to go find work). Actually, I
lie. I'm not in Mexico. In fact, I've never even been to Mexico, because
if I want to suffer diarrhea for a week, I can do it much more cheaply by
just visiting my mom.

So, to be honest, this chapter on alcohol was written, as were all the
other chapters, in my home and at my desk, and it thus presented a
huge challenge because as a "method writer" I tried to write as much of
this chapter as I could by getting into the spirit of it, as it were, so if

some of what you read here doesn't sound to you quite as coherent as the rest of the book, then you'll know why.

This chapter was also, to borrow a word from my son, the McGill English major, the funnest (well, McGill is in French-speaking Montreal, after all) to work on. I think it may be the funnest one for you to read, too, because my advice while you're reading this stuff is to take a page from the author and become a "method" reader, and drink, drink, drink (well, maybe you should stop at two drinks) while reading it.

Anyway, as the urologists always say in the OR just before making the first cut, "*Cin, cin.*" Just kidding, guys, so don't look so worried. Way more often, it's actually "*L'Chaim,*" at least among the urologists I know.

Is Alcohol Good for You?

This won't surprise anyone who knows me or who has read anything I've written before, but for the one or two of you being introduced to my fine writing for the first time, I must tell you that I firmly believe that *for most people, the benefits of alcohol significantly outweigh the risks* and that drinking moderate amounts of alcohol regularly is a very healthy thing for most of us to do, certainly on a par with (and perhaps even better than) following a healthy diet and probably even on a par with taking widely prescribed and very useful drugs such as cholesterol-lowering medications.

Yes, I know that most of the positive findings about alcohol come from observational studies, and as stated earlier, it's possible to go drastically wrong in such studies, by either misreading the variables or being seduced by observer bias.

Nevertheless, I doubt that these potential sources of error account for the multitude of positive findings about alcohol—the evidence is just too thick that a moderate intake of alcohol is good for most of us. I'm going to present the other side, too, but for the moment, let's stick with the good stuff.

WHICH FORM OF ALCOHOL IS BEST?

Actually, that's hard to say.

In support of the brew overwhelmingly favored by those who still hit each other on the heads with bones and pirate the losers' mates, an Israeli study concluded that drinking 340 milliliters (12 fluid ounces) of beer for a month led to positive changes in blood lipid levels and to a reduced ability of the blood to clot, both of which should eventually lead to fewer heart attacks. Although I must say that when I first read it, I pooh-poohed this study because of the obvious: what do Jewish researchers know about drinking beer, anyway? I mean, I could easily accept a study from Israel about the benefits of Manischewitz Concord grape wine (Concord wine is great for marinating a brisket, by the way), but a study about beer? Gimme a break.

I was somewhat mollified, however, when I learned that a Dutch study came to exactly the same conclusion as the Israeli study. Those people in the North Country do know something about beer, so there may really be something to this connection between beer and better health. Those findings aside, however, I believe that wine probably pips beer or grain alcohol, though this belief may have a lot to do with the fact that I'm not allowed to drink beer or many alcoholic drinks. My allergy to gluten, which is found in barley, means that if I drink beer, I not only get sick but also raise my risk of developing lymphoma, and believe me, no Corona is worth a cancer.

Whatever the reason, though, I favor a mellow merlot or a perky pinot noir over a classy chardonnay and especially over a classless Coors, because I believe that there's enough evidence to conclude that red wine is probably the best alcoholic drink to consume. I have no idea if it's due to the resveratrol in the wine, the polyphenols, the flavonoids, or the phytoalexins, or even to the delicious and flavorful nitric oxide synthesase, all of which are important components of red wine that have been linked to health benefits (some are present in white wine, too, but usually in lower amounts). In the end, it may even just be the prettier color of great red wines, but overall I'm convinced that red wine has more benefits than beer or white wine.

Indeed, some researchers recently declared that there may even be a qualitative difference among red wines. These guys concluded that red wine from France is much more healthful than red wine from Germany, and the real surprise is that it was German researchers, not French researchers, who came to that conclusion. If you ask me, this only demonstrates the depth to which this current generation of Germans is willing to dive to help forge a new Franco-German anti-American alliance.

◆ ——————————————————————————————— ◆

A FEW DEFINITIONS

What do we mean by "light," "moderate," and "heavy" alcohol intake? To answer this question we must first define what a "standard drink" is.

A *standard drink* is generally defined as 12 grams (0.42 ounces) of alcohol, which is found in:

- A single 340-milliliter (12-fluid-ounce) can of beer (and please note, football fans, that's a small can of beer).
- One 142-milliliter (5-fluid-ounce) glass of wine. Again, please note that's a small glass of wine. I've been in homes where they pour 227-milliliter (8-fluid-ounce) glasses of wine, though never *chez moi;* as a considerate host, I tend to pour my guests 57-milliliter (2-fluid-ounce) glasses, and phooey on all those who say that's just because I'm cheap. Besides, my wife isn't paying for that stuff.
- 43 milliliters (1.5 fluid ounces) of 80-proof alcohol.

Light alcohol intake generally consists of drinking *one or fewer* of those standard drinks every day or several times a week.

Moderate intake is generally defined as a daily dose of *two to three of those measures.* (Some Europeans, however, especially French researchers, consider anything up to four units a day to still be within the limits of "moderate" intake, which is why I love visiting France.) Alternately, in North America, it is usually recommended that to stick to moderate amounts of intake, women drink no more than nine units a week and men drink 14 or fewer units a week.

Heavy alcohol intake is generally accepted to be *four or more* standard alcohol drinks over a 24-hour period.

But as always, it's not that simple. The numbers tell only part of the story, because in determining the health benefits from alcohol intake, you also have to take into account *how a drinker drinks his booze.* "But there is only one way to drink booze," I can hear some of the slow readers who are now into their third glass of wine protesting. Well, you're wrong, *mon ami;* there is more than one way to drain a chard. There is moderate drinking, and then there is binge-drinking—defined as five or more drinks in one sitting—and binge-drinking is very bad for your health (see below). Someone who binges, say, three times a week can still manage to average less than that 21-drink limit that's generally accepted as the definition of moderate alcohol intake, yet his or her health would be very adversely affected.

◆ ──────────────────────────────── ◆

DO WE ALL BENEFIT FROM ALCOHOL?

Something that often gets lost in the storm of glad findings about alcohol is that we are not all equally likely to benefit from drinking alcohol regularly.

To start, no study has even shown that someone who doesn't drink alcohol and who feels healthy despite his lack of a life (just kidding— I'm sure that people who drink only herbal tea do indeed lead quite fascinating lives, but they're so mellow, who would ever know?) would help themselves much by starting to drink alcohol. So mark this down: there is *no evidence to support getting a teetotaler to start drinking,* or for that matter, for anyone to move from being a light drinker to a moderate drinker.

Another important point: adolescents have far more to lose than to gain from drinking even small amounts of alcohol regularly.

What might surprise you to learn, though, is that young midlifers also have less to gain from drinking alcohol than older midlifers. So it's likely that a man or woman of 40, say, has far more to gain from other health adjustments than from boozing.

It's only when you get well up in middle age that the benefits of alcohol really kick in, because that's when you start having major risks for the kind of damage alcohol might protect you from.

One study tried to quantify the benefits of drinking alcohol and concluded that because the benefits kick in later in life, males should not start drinking until they reach age 34 and females should not drink until age 54. I tried to point this out to my young son one time, but he cynically suggested that I just wanted to keep all the booze to myself. Smart kid.

Finally, there are certain people who should *avoid alcohol at all times*, including:

- Pregnant women
- People with known drinking problems
- People with a family history of alcoholism
- People with chronic conditions such as liver disease
- People on many different types of medication
- People with a history of substance abuse

Specific Health Benefits

HEART

Moderate alcohol consumption is at least as effective as, and probably more effective than, diet, drugs, or any other protective mechanisms you can name in protecting your heart, with the exceptions of giving up cigarettes and perhaps exercise.

A recent update of the Health Professionals Follow-Up Study concluded that any kind of regular alcohol-drinking reduces the risk of heart attack. However, this study is really bad news for the more-is-always-better-when-it-comes-to-the-good-things-in-life crowd, because it found that only a bit of alcohol (one drink three to four days a week) was the optimal level for lowering the risk of heart attack, an amount that is less than most other studies have determined as the optimum intake.

But, you may say, an American male health professional is not exactly representative of a typical member of society, and I agree with you. Not only are we talking about some majorly weird folks, we're also talking about a group of guys who are generally much better off than the average person and who probably do more to stay healthy than does the average man (although if, like me, you've seen far too many male health professionals and especially physicians with their clothes off — in the OR dressing room only, I hasten to add — you might wonder how much these guys really do to stay healthy).

So let me tell you about a group of guys who are probably more like the average beer-drinking, nacho-noshing male reader of this book: overweight middle-aged Danish men with abnormal lipid levels, whose sole idea of exercise probably consists of lifting another herring or schnapps to their mouths. These men also have fewer heart attacks if they drink moderate amounts of alcohol than a similar group of Hamlets who don't drink alcohol regularly. Same thing was found in a study from Honolulu, which has been tracking the health of male residents of Paradise for many years, and in a study from the Netherlands, another from Britain, one from Italy, one from China, and on and on. So this alcohol-is-good-for-the-male-heart stuff is pretty international.

What about women? The Nurses' Health Study found that, just as for men, moderate women drinkers have about half the rate of heart attacks as do nondrinkers. The really great thing about this study is that it ruled out potential interfering factors such as diet, body build, smoking, and exercise, yet that pro-alcohol finding still held. Even in a crowd of women who were all slim healthy eaters, regular exercisers, and nonsmokers, regular drinkers of alcohol ended up with significantly fewer heart attacks than nondrinkers. (How in the world they found enough slim, healthy-eating, nonsmoking, exercising nurses to fill out that side of the study, I'll never know, unless, of course, nurses have changed a whole lot from the time I was in training, when Nurse Ratched was my unit supervisor.)

Finally, you know whose hearts might actually gain the most from drinking alcohol regularly? People who've already had one heart attack. A study found that men who've suffered a heart attack and who subsequently drink alcohol have about half the rate of a second heart attack as teetotalers. These results are so impressive that one might be sorely tempted to recommend that anyone who's had a heart attack take up drinking alcohol even before they swallow their first ASA (but one really doesn't have the guts to make that recommendation, does one?).

And how does alcohol benefit the heart?

I once read the following headline in the *Onion*, a satirical webzine: *Report: Aspirin taken daily with fifth of bourbon reduces awareness of heart attacks.* I'm sure that's true, though I've never seen it proved in a study.

On a more practical level, alcohol:

• Lowers LDL levels and raises HDL levels, especially after fatty meals, when you really need that benefit to kick in.

- Affects several enzymes that help thin the blood, thus making it less likely to clot.
- Improves the body's ability to deal with blood sugar, thus lowering the eventual risk of diabetes.
- Lowers the level of inflammation in the cardiovascular system (see chapter 1) and elsewhere.
- May lower blood pressure. It's been hard to get consensus on the exact effect of moderate alcohol intake on blood pressure, though at least one good study of young adults found the lowest blood pressures in those who drank moderate amounts of alcohol regularly.
- Contains a number of antioxidants, those enzymes that mop up free radicals and help keep the body younger and disease-free.
- Is a wonderful—and cheap—product to improve mood and lower stress and anxiety levels, something that rarely gets the attention I think it deserves. (What, me worry about the kids, Phyllis? You handle it; I'll have another glass of wine.)
- Is a reward that makes all the other healthy lifestyle practices worth doing. The payoff of being allowed to drink a glass or two of wine every night is often what keeps me doing as much exercise as I do.
- Increases estrogen levels. Ever notice, guys, how you urgently want to redecorate the playroom and call your sister to chat after having a couple of drinks? You haven't? Well, you're the exception, I assure you.

STROKE

Alcohol also lowers the risk of some kinds of stroke. Specifically, people who drink moderate amounts of alcohol tend to have fewer ischemic strokes (the most common form of stroke, caused by a blockage in a blood vessel) than do nondrinkers.

But drinking even moderate amounts of alcohol raises the risk of hemorrhagic strokes, those caused by a bleed into the brain (see below).

BRAIN

A recent large Swedish study concluded that elderly men and women who drink on average two or fewer alcoholic drinks a day have lower levels of dementia than do nondrinkers.

This is not a new finding, by the way, since several other studies have found the same thing. For example, a study from Japan found that midlife Japanese who drank moderate amounts of wine or saki did better on IQ tests than did teetotalers and heavy drinkers, and an American study on elderly nurses found that those who drank moderate amounts of alcohol regularly did better on tests of brain function—their brains were said to be "one to two years younger"—than did women who didn't drink or who drank too much. And a more than 20-year Danish study found that midlifers who drank moderate amounts of wine regularly ended up with half the rate of dementia of a comparable group of abstainers, though those who drank beer regularly were not similarly protected.

So it's commonly accepted now that regular moderate alcohol drinkers are less likely to develop dementia than others. Of course, it could simply be that elderly people who drink regularly are more likely to have lived healthier lives so they start with healthier brains compared to nondrinkers, but hey, I prefer to think that alcohol actually helps the brain.

How does alcohol protect brain cells? It's probably just more of the same old, same old. Alcohol:

- Improves blood flow in blood vessels.
- Improves lipid levels.
- Lowers the blood's ability to clot.
- Contains antioxidants.
- Has an anti-inflammatory effect.
- Might even help tissues repair themselves.
- Lowers the risk of stroke (see above), which may also proffer a secondary advantage to the brain, because some types of dementia are now associated with multiple tiny ischemic strokes, so lowering the risk of strokes also lowers the eventual risk of dementia.

Other Benefits
Common diseases and conditions that may be ameliorated or in part prevented by drinking moderate amounts of alcohol regularly include:

- *Diabetes.* Studies have found that men and especially women who drink moderate amounts of alcohol have better control of their blood glucose and hence lower risks of Type 2 diabetes.
- *Cancer.* One study found that red wine may help stop prostate cancer cells from proliferating. Another found that men who consumed the highest amounts of boron (which happens to be plentiful in red wine) were also much less likely than their boron-barren brothers to develop prostate cancer. Although I'd never advise you to protect your prostate by downing Chateau Roth-gut every night, if you do happen to enjoy the odd glass, you can rest easier that it may also be doing you some good where the sun don't shine. Wine drinkers may also have lower risks of *non-Hodgkin's lymphoma,* one of the most rapidly increasing malignancies in North America.
- *Absenteeism.* In Finland, people who drink small to moderate amounts of alcohol regularly lose less work than do teetotaling Finns. ("Why are you drinking, Petri?"; "Because I really want to go to work tomorrow, Jyrki.")
- *Osteoporosis.*
- *Hearing loss.*
- *Erectile dysfunction.*
- *Colds and flus.* You get fewer colds when you drink alcohol regularly, and besides, even if you get a cold, it doesn't feel as bad after a couple of hot toddies.
- *Macular degeneration.*
- *Gallstones.*
- *Hospitalization* for any cause (though this benefit must, of course, be weighed against the huge number of hospitalizations as a result of excess alcohol intake).
- *Disability* in old age.
- *Hepatitis A.*
- *Rheumatoid arthritis.*
- *Gastritis and ulcers.* Regular alcohol intake may lower the risk of ulcer because alcohol protects the stomach against infection from the bacteria known as *Helicobacter pylori,* the most common cause of ulcer.

Drawbacks

So that's the good stuff, but like so many other things in life, such as ABBA, military intervention in the Middle East, and especially the Germans, alcohol is difficult to endorse unreservedly, since it can also cost people's health and their lives. (Listening to ABBA for hours on end—as one of my sons used to make me do—doesn't ruin your physical health; it just plays havoc with your mental well-being). The benefits of alcohol are not always obvious or accepted by everyone, but its drawbacks are grave and clear and numerous.

DRUNKENNESS

I know this is obvious, but it's really worth stating clearly: alcohol gets you drunk and alters your mental state. Becoming drunk and the changes it leads to are influenced by several very important factors:

- Speed kills. The faster, you drink, the higher your peak blood alcohol concentration goes. In layman's English that means if you chug, say, four beers in a few minutes, you're going to hit a higher blood alcohol level (often much higher) than if you drink those four beers over the space of a few hours. I know that for many of you this is one of those *duhhhhh! geee!* kind of observations, but hey, to a chugging college stud, that information may come as a surprise.
- Eating slows down the rate of absorption of any alcohol you're consuming at the same time, though not nearly as much as most of us want to believe it does.
- Size matters. All else being equal, basketball pylon Yao Ming can put away a lot more alcohol than Pee Wee Hister before it starts to affect him, because larger people have a larger volume of blood, and a larger blood volume dilutes alcohol more than a smaller volume.
- Increasing alcohol intake results in gradually increasing tolerance to alcohol. The more you drink, the more alcohol it eventually takes to give you the same effect, which is why anyone who's a heavy drinker will take longer and require greater amounts of alcohol to get drunk than someone like me, who is much more sparing in his alcohol intake.

- Pre-existing mood and psychological state can influence how alcohol effects a drinker. If you are depressed or anxious, for example, alcohol is likely to accentuate those states, whereas if you drink when you're more upbeat, then alcohol is likely to produce a more euphoric effect. Also, according to a recent study, people who are quick to get angry are significantly more likely to become aggressive if they drink too much than less anger-prone individuals are. And if you're tired or sleep-deprived, alcohol's effects on those states are likely to be exaggerated, too.

  Then there's this curious finding: a study from New Zealand concluded that being drunk is at least partly "in the mind," meaning that people who think they're going to get drunk tend to act and behave more drunk on smaller amounts of alcohol than people who don't believe they're going to get drunk. In this ingenious study, two groups of students were given tonic water to drink, but the students in one group were told they were drinking vodka and that they were drunk from its effects (clearly, none of them were A students, but then again, maybe they were). These students had poorer memories for learned facts and tended to be much more suggestible (both of which are signs of being drunk) than the students who had been told the truth.

- Research has also found that some people experience more of a stimulating and hence euphoric effect from alcohol than others; the former are more likely to drink excessively to attain that feeling more often than is good for them.

- Women can't handle booze as easily as men, so women generally tend to show visible signs of alcohol intoxication (sidling up to the loser in the cutoff T-shirt at the bar, for example, or telling her best friend that she had an affair with her husband, though women often do stuff like that even when they're not drunk) at much lower levels of alcohol intake than do men.

  What's wrong with women? Wait, let me rephrase that. Why are women not able to consume as much alcohol as men without showing visible signs of intoxication? For one thing, women lack an enzyme (alcohol dehydrogenase) in their livers and stomachs that breaks alcohol down, so, measure for measure, much more alcohol reaches women's bloodstreams than men's. Thus, women tend to get more drunk and stay drunk longer on smaller volumes of alcohol than do men.

In addition, because women are not as large as men on average, they have a smaller volume of blood in which to dilute alcohol. It has also been claimed that a high level of testosterone might allow a man to drink a lot of alcohol without becoming as intoxicated as someone who has much less circulating testosterone. In contrast, however, higher levels of estrogen (and other female hormones) might result in a relatively poor ability to metabolize alcohol.

- Certain racial groups also lack some of the enzymes needed to break down alcohol, so members of those groups, too, get drunk at lower levels of alcohol intake.
- Bingeing is probably the worst way to drink alcohol. For a start, binge drinkers are much more likely to get much more drunk than are regular, more restrained alcohol users. Binge-drinking is also associated disproportionately with impaired judgment (see below). To underline how bad the judgment of binge drinkers is, one survey revealed that nearly 75 percent of binge drinkers consider themselves to be "moderate drinkers," meaning they think they're getting the health benefits of alcohol because they consume less than 21 units a week. But let me ask you this: would you really be protecting your teeth if you brushed them 14 times on Saturday, and then did nothing for the rest of the week, because, hey, after all, you would still be averaging brushing your teeth twice a day for the full week? It's the same with drinking alcohol: the average is not nearly as important in many instances as the matter of how the drinker got there.

Worst of all, binge drinkers are at far greater risk of premature death as a result of their alcohol intake than teetotalers or moderate drinkers who limit themselves to two glasses of quality claret nightly before shuffling off to their well-deserved repose.

Some experts estimate that binge-drinking accounts for over half the annual deaths attributable to alcohol. Binge drinkers not only have much higher risks of heart attacks and strokes than moderate drinkers do, but are also 14 times as likely to drink and drive and are much more likely to be killed in motor vehicle accidents, industrial accidents, suicides, and homicides, as well as other forms of violent death (not to mention that they're also much more likely to kill others, of course).

Finally, binge drinkers are also much more likely than social drinkers to be attacked by someone in a bar who's had enough of hearing "Help Me Make It Through the Night" played on the jukebox for the 11th straight time.

What's really worrisome is that binge-drinking has become much more "in." A recent American study found that more than 25 percent of the population has been involved in at least one episode of binge-drinking over the preceding 12 months, an increase of over 35 percent since 1996. Yes, this is undoubtedly in part a reflection of what's happening on our college campuses. (During the horrendous ice storm that hit Montreal a few years ago, I was concerned when the water was cut off in my son's dormitory at McGill. "Don't worry, Dad," he reassured me. "We have lots of beer." Silly me for worrying!) But in this survey, over 70 percent of binge drinkers were over the age of 25, and even my son, he of the eight-year B.A. program, is not likely to be a college undergraduate at the age of 26, at least I hope not.

In addition, according to most surveys, young women are beginning to engage in binge-drinking in much larger numbers than ever before. Indeed, in some parts of the world, binge-drinking among young women is now as common as it is among young men. A British survey found that significantly more young women in the U.K. are now binge-drinking at least once a week, that one-third of twenty-something females admit to having unprotected sex while drunk, and that 57 percent of women under the age of 24 admitted that on occasion they've been so drunk they had no memory of the night before (my wife often says that, too, and she doesn't even drink; I think that's called wishful thinking). What's more, these women not only drink too much and fool around too much, they also fight more; 14 percent of these binge-drinking women also admitted to having a fistfight while drunk.

MORTALITY

Excess alcohol kills. American public health officials attribute over 100,000 deaths a year directly to alcohol intake, making it the third leading cause of preventable death after smoking and lack of activity.

Excess alcohol intake can kill you in many ways. A major Scandinavian review of heavy drinking patterns found that people who consume large amounts of alcohol (whether bingeing or by slow accumulation) have a significantly increased risk of dying from:

- Heart attacks
- Strokes
- Other cardiovascular problems
- Accidents
- Violent deaths
- Gastrointestinal diseases
- Certain cancers, such as liver cancer and breast cancer

UNSUCCESSFUL AGING

In the Harvard Study of Adult Development, the third best predictor (after not smoking and having good coping skills) of "successful" aging (making the transition into becoming an older person in a healthy and happy manner) was *not drinking to excess*. This is not the only study to have come to the same conclusion: drinking to excess not only ages you prematurely as a result of tissue breakdown and disease but also hurts you emotionally, financially, spiritually, and socially and greatly handicaps your ability to successfully manage the often difficult passage into old age. Of course, if you don't want to live to a happy old age, then...

EFFECTS ON THE BRAIN AND NERVOUS SYSTEM

Alcohol has adverse effects on the brain in many varied ways.

Judgment

Even small amounts of alcohol cloud judgment, though clearly, the more you drink, the worse the decisions you tend to make—something scientists refer to as the "beer-goggle" effect. This is best illustrated by those times when an otherwise thoughtful, careful woman wakes up next to Quasimodo when the previous night she was certain she was bedding George Clooney. (I met my wife, by the way, on one of the few nights in my life when I got blindly drunk—they were giving away free beer to medical students. She was, as always, completely sober, so the moral, she says, is that being sober can also cloud your judgment. She's kidding, of course.)

The really sad thing is that it doesn't take much alcohol to get that beer-goggle giggle going. According to one study, a blood alcohol level of .04 percent, about half the legal limit in many provinces and states (usually reached in men after two small glasses of wine or two beers, and less in women), was enough to leave many people unaware that they were making errors of judgment in specially contrived tests.

Ordinarily, you see, when you make a mistake, you recognize right away that you've made an error (unless, of course, your name is Bill Clinton); it's the so-called "oops" response. But in this study, people who drank even small amounts of alcohol not only made the expected larger number of mistakes, but also had lots more trouble recognizing that they'd made those mistakes. These findings were confirmed by brain scans that showed that the "oops" center was indeed much slower than normal to charge into action after even very small amounts of alcohol. Thus, if you're driving drunk, not only are you more likely to swerve into oncoming traffic or drive onto the shoulder or run a red light, you're also less likely to recognize that you just made those errors, so you are even slower than you would otherwise have been to correct those potentially lethal mistakes.

Coordination
This needs little explaining; any amount of alcohol quickly impairs co-ordination and reaction time, and the more you drink, the worse the impairment.

Brain Cell Death
There is apparently no basis to the widely held belief that any alcohol intake at all kills brain cells. After all, just look at this long-time moderate alcohol consumer. Well, maybe I should offer stronger support to that argument: Walter Hunt, Ph.D., a senior science advisor at the

National Institute on Alcohol Abuse and Alcoholism (NIAAA) was quoted in an article for *WebMD Health* as saying, "There is presently no strong evidence to conclude that any given session of alcohol consumption causes brain cells to die."

However, chronic heavy use of alcohol does *kill brain cells*, including centers in the frontal lobes involved in emotions and some higher brain functions, such as planning and attention. No surprise, then, that one study found that the brains of alcoholic women were 11 percent smaller than the brains of nondrinking women. One startling way in which alcohol affects the brain is through its role in malnutrition (see below). For example, chronic alcohol intake commonly leads to deficiencies in vitamin B1, and this in turn leads to a condition known as Korsakoff's syndrome, which affects memory, especially the ability to retain new information. We used to see this syndrome only in older alcoholics, but sadly, in western Scotland, researchers report a significant rise in the number of young women with Korsakoff's syndrome because of binge-drinking (though the Brits insist on calling it Korsakov's syndrome; maybe Korsakoff defected, or maybe he consulted a numerologist), and I'm sure Scotland is not unique in this regard.

Memory

Excess alcohol intake has long been known to damage what is known as retrospective memory, that is, memory of past events—as, for example, "Did I eat an hour ago?" But a recent study found that drinking too much alcohol negatively affects "prospective" memory, too, that is, remembering to do things in the future—as, for example, "I must remember to eat in an hour."

Mental health

Heavy alcohol use is also associated with all sorts of psychological problems, including chronic anxiety, panic attacks, and especially depression, though for many heavy drinkers it's hard to say which came first, the psychological problem or the alcohol abuse. But excess alcohol intake will always make a mental health problem worse, which is especially sad because lots of people clearly attempt to self-medicate their psychological conditions with alcohol.

Stroke

Although, as stated previously, moderate alcohol intake lowers the risk of that form of stroke known as ischemic stroke, this is at least partly offset by the fact that any alcohol intake at all increases the risk of the less common form of stroke known as a hemorrhagic stroke, which is caused by the rupture of a blood vessel. That's because alcohol helps prevent clotting, so when a blood vessel develops a small tear, say, or some other weak point, one that could naturally heal with a clot, alcohol lowers the tendency for such a clot to form.

As well, chronic heavy alcohol use significantly raises the risk of both types of stroke.

EFFECTS ON THE HEART AND BLOOD VESSELS

Alcohol excess can have several deleterious effects on the heart and blood vessels. First, it's been estimated that alcohol abuse accounts for anywhere from 5 to 20 percent of all cases of high blood pressure in North America. Alcohol abuse also raises the risks of heart attack, cardiac rhythm abnormalities, and inappropriate growth of the heart (you want a big heart, but not too big, because then it stops working properly).

EFFECTS ON THE LIVER

They get little attention, but together cirrhosis and liver disease are the 10th leading cause of death in North America, and by far the leading contributor to liver damage is heavy use of alcohol. Liver disease, by the way, does not just manifest itself with hepatitis, fatty liver, and cirrhosis; liver damage can also lead to liver cancer, clotting abnormalities, immune system malfunctioning, and poor absorption of many vitamins.

CANCER

Alcohol is known to raise the risk of several cancers, including:

- *Breast cancer.* According to an excellent review in the *British Journal of Cancer*, alcohol raises the risk of breast cancer in women with every drink taken; every extra glass of wine consumed as a daily average raises the risk of breast cancer by 6 percent. For overall health, however, the benefits of alcohol in reducing the risk of heart disease still outweigh the risk of breast cancer, especially for women who are several years past menopause, when the rate of death from heart disease starts to climb sharply. Given how frightening the prospect of breast cancer is for most women, however, each woman has to make her own call on this one. The risk of breast cancer from alcohol is compounded by the use of hormone replacement therapy (HRT) for menopause (I sincerely hope that most women are not taking HRT any longer, but that risk can be reduced by taking folic acid [see chapter 4]).

- *Lung cancer.* The very high risks of lung cancer (as well as other oral and upper respiratory cancers) that smokers face are made even higher if smokers drink alcohol to excess.
- *Other cancers.* Cancers of the pharynx, liver, esophagus, and colon and rectum, among others, are more common in heavy drinkers.

Animal studies also indicate that heavy alcohol use may be a cancer accelerator; that is, alcohol might speed up the rate at which malignancies develop and the rate at which they turn nasty.

MALNUTRITION
Chronic alcohol abuse goes hand-in-hand with poor eating habits. In addition, alcohol interferes with the absorption of certain nutrients (vitamins, calcium, zinc) and with the normal metabolism of other nutrients (especially folic acid). The result is that chronic alcoholics are often very malnourished individuals.

VIOLENCE
I'm not going to belabor this, because surely you already know it. People who can't handle alcohol and who drink too much are very, very, very disproportionately involved in:

- Random acts of violence
- Sexual abuse
- Domestic violence
- Motor vehicle injuries

- Falls
- Arson
- Accidents
- Homicides
- Industrial injuries

Drinking is so intimately related to accidents that people who have been drinking are significantly more likely than nondrinkers to suffer severe head injuries when involved in a motor vehicle accident—even when they're passengers.

EFFECTS ON SLEEP

Although many of us think of alcohol as a sleep inducer (every woman I know looks as if she's ready to nod off after two sips of wine, which may not tell you as much about alcohol as it does about the women I know, or the men who try to keep them up), excess alcohol actually interferes with sleep. Never use alcohol as a sleep aid, even though, as we all know, lots of people do.

EFFECTS ON WEIGHT

Alcohol contains 7 calories per gram, and as a general rule, a standard glass of alcohol contributes nearly 100 calories to your daily load. So it stands to reason that drinking any alcohol at all should lead to weight gain. In fact, a recent review in the *American Journal of Clinical Nutrition* that tracked over 6,800 British middle-aged men for five years concluded that they gained weight directly in proportion to the amount they drank.

Yes, but.

Yes, but it also depends a lot on how much and what you eat. For example, if you've ever had the mixed pleasure of seeing a beached, bikinied, baking, beer-slurping male stripped to the waist, you might at first attribute those rolls and that beer belly entirely to his alcohol intake. But that Moby is also very likely to have a poor diet (witness the several hot dogs and bags of fries he's consumed as you've watched him), and he's also very unlikely to be doing any exercise, and those factors may have more to do with why he's now being approached by two worried Greenpeace workers than does his alcohol intake. If, however, a moderate consumer of alcohol also exercises and eats well, it's unlikely that the alcohol intake would have much effect on his or her weight.

Some people, on the other hand, clearly do gain lots of weight from their drinking. This may have something to do with their genes. Italian scientists recently linked a gene called DD (wasn't she a Mouseketeer?) that's present in about 40 percent of the population with excessive weight around the abdomen caused by alcohol intake (in Italian, *beero belliano*), and as you no doubt remember from chapter 1, this is a particularly bad place to lay down your extra pounds.

INTERACTIONS WITH MEDICATIONS

Alcohol interacts with and interferes with many medications. For example, it can lead to life-threatening liver damage when taken with acetaminophen (better known to many of you as Tylenol), and in some people this has apparently happened with as few as one to two drinks and two acetaminophen tablets.

Alcohol is doubly and triply dangerous when it's taken with certain psychoactive drugs, such as tranquilizers and antidepressants, and with any other drugs that can produce drowsiness, such as antihistamines. The combination of many drugs with alcohol can lead to nausea, vomiting, fainting, and even cardiac abnormalities. Alcohol can also cause the drug you're taking to be much less effective.

If you're taking medications, always check carefully to make sure that your drugs are compatible with your level of alcohol intake. With some drugs, such as tranquilizers, you're probably best off avoiding any drinking at all.

USE WITH RECREATIONAL DRUGS

Studies have shown that those of you who enjoy combining alcohol with marijuana (usually ugly fat men with ponytails who call everyone "Man" or "Dude") have a much greater chance of seriously injuring yourselves than if you (ab)use either substance alone. Bummer, dude.

EFFECTS ON TESTOSTERONE

According to a recent study in rats, alcohol leads to a surge of testosterone in the brain, though some human studies have shown that alcohol leads to a drop in levels of testosterone circulating in the blood. So the bottom line, I guess, is that some men who drink excessively will find that one morning they've joined the Marines, while others will find they've married the girl they never meant to marry, or perhaps even become the girl they never meant to become.

EFFECTS DURING PREGNANCY

There is no known safe amount of alcohol for pregnant women to consume if they want to protect their unborn babies from the potentially awful consequences of fetal alcohol syndrome. Recent studies suggest that even moderate amounts of alcohol during pregnancy may leave babies with subtle developmental and emotional defects.

Pregnant women who drink also raise the risk their baby will die of SIDS (sudden infant death syndrome). One study found that the female children of women who drink while pregnant have a greater risk of developing behavior problems later in life, another found that the children of women who drank while pregnant had a higher risk of breast cancer as adults, while yet another found that babies born to women who drink while pregnant are three times as likely to end up alcoholics themselves as are the kids of nondrinking moms.

So, pregnant women shouldn't drink any alcohol at all. Period. Sadly, however, a recent study found that up to 15 percent of women still drink alcohol during their pregnancy, and 6 percent reported at least one binge episode while pregnant. Given that people always downplay their negative habits when answering surveys, you can safely assume that the real numbers are higher, which is sad news, I think.

OTHER PHYSICAL EFFECTS

And if all that's not enough for you, excess alcohol intake is also associated with increased risks of:

- Diabetes
- Pancreatitis
- Age-related maculopathy
- Gout
- Hypoglycemia in diabetics
- Kidney disease and kidney failure
- Neuropathies

And just to add insult to major injury, the *heaviest drinkers also tend to be the heaviest smokers.*

SOCIAL EFFECTS

Effects on family and friends

Often the saddest consequence of chronic heavy use of alcohol is the devastating effect on the family and friends of the drinker, which often sets them up for physical, psychiatric, psychological, and social problems. It is said that on average an alcoholic has a significant negative effect on five other people.

◆ ———————————————————— ◆

WHAT TO DO IF YOU THINK YOU HAVE A DRINKING PROBLEM

Even if you just think you have an alcohol problem, you have an alcohol problem, and there are only two things to do:

- Admit it openly.
- Ask for help.

The first one is the harder of the two, but once you've done it, it leads naturally to the second.

As to specific therapies, try any one (family docs, counselors, special programs) that you think fits your personality and state, though I will urge you, no matter what else you try, to at least give Alcoholics Anonymous a shot (no pun intended). According to a recent report in the journal *Alcoholism: Clinical and Experimental Research,* alcoholics who attended AA were three times as likely to stay sober over the long term than those who did not obtain support or who got support other than from AA.

What's so special about AA? I have never been to AA (though on one of my early-morning walks to the TV studio I was once accosted by someone who asked if I was on my way to an AA meeting, which may reveal a bit about what I look like at 8 AM), so I don't really know what goes on there. The study's researchers don't seem to know what's so special about AA, either.

They do say that it's not the well-known spirituality of AA that accounts for its effectiveness, because the most spiritual AA attendees do no better at staying off drinking than the less spiritual members. But whatever it is that AA does, it works. In fact, this report found that even those AA members who were going outside AA to get help for their drinking still relied on AA as backup.

◆ ——————————————————————————————————— ◆

Effects on parenting

Every time I see my father staring back at me in the mirror I thank God he was so bloody good-looking, but I am also forced to admit that there's clearly a large genetic component to our lives that we just can't escape. I mean, that's Henry Hister in the mirror, folks, not me. How did that happen? And at such a young age?

But our parents also exert a subtle—and stronger—influence than that imposed by our genes only. That is also why every time I yell at my kids, I hear my dad yelling at me. We learn a lot about how to behave from patterns our parents taught us, so it's no surprise, for example, that the sons and daughters of smokers are much more likely to end up smokers than are the kids of nonsmokers.

There is certainly a strong genetic component to alcohol abuse, but there's also a strong parental environmental influence. Thus, kids who watch their parents abusing alcohol are much more likely to end up seduced by demon Drambuie themselves. As well, parents who drink heavily are much more likely to be neglectful parents and so children of heavy drinkers are more likely to have behavior problems, to abuse drugs and alcohol, and to be involved in high-risk behavior than the kids of people who use alcohol more wisely.

CHAPTER

7

Smoking

Watch Your Butts

Smoking is one of the leading causes of statistics.
FLETCHER KNEBEL

One thousand Americans stop smoking every day—
by dying.
AUTHOR UNKNOWN

IF IT WERE UP TO ME, I wouldn't write more than four words about smoking in this book. To wit: "If you smoke, stop." Make that five words: "If you smoke, stop, dummy." But my contract stipulates that I must write an entire chapter on smoking—a topic that I believe has been done to death (much like, heh, heh, what smoking does to smokers, of course).

"But why do the publisher and the author have such divergent opinions about the need for lots of information about smoking in this book?" you might wonder.

Well, it's really quite simple, at least according to the author. The publisher probably still sends letters to the North Pole every Christmas and donates to Greenpeace. That's all that could explain, the author believes, the publisher's firmly stated opinion that there are still lots of smokers out there who need only be pointed in the right direction to take the proffered bit by their rotting and discolored teeth and do the right thing and give up their noxious and toxic habit.

In contrast, the author does not believe that anything he says is going to matter a whit to a smoker. I once gave a speech about living a healthy lifestyle to a group of army vets—the hardest room I've ever worked, by the way; the only time they briefly perked their ears up was when I discussed the health benefits of drinking alcohol, and that was only to interrupt me with salutations and toasts, a barrage of "Think I'll have one more, Doc" and "Here's to you, Doc."

Anyway, after the talk, I was approached by a grizzled, bent-over, medal-bedecked gent in a blue uniform (I thought at first he was a con-cessionaire), who said he was a veteran who was "over 70, Sonny, but I look much younger, eh?" To which the answer was clearly no, but I de-murred. He went on to inform me that he and all his mates had smoked their "entire lives" (I had to suppress a giggle at the image of a smoking infant, though in the Canadian army, hey, who knows?) and that he was living proof that I was dead wrong about the hazards of smoking. See? Smoking had done nothing harmful to him, so there.

"And your friends?" I asked innocently, waving my arm at the room. "They're well, too?"

"Hell, no," he said. "These are not my real friends. All my real friends are dead."

He stood there for a moment with a triumphant smile on his face (though I suppose it could also have been gas), then left. For once, I was speechless. I tell you this story because it clearly shows that smokers are as dense as gym mats—something that science readily confirms, by the way, or as Mona Lisa Vito says in *My Cousin Vinny*, "It's a fact." For example, one American survey revealed that nearly three-quarters of women smokers claimed that they were not aware that they had the same risk of getting lung cancer as do men smokers. I mean, *duuuhhh!*

Over 50 percent of these women smokers were also not aware that they were at much higher risk of developing heart disease as a result of their filthy habit. Double *duhhh!* I mean, that's dumb.

And lest you get the wrong idea, I don't for an instant mean to imply that women smokers are dumber than men smokers, because hey, men are always at least as dumb as women. Men smokers are morons, too.

By the way, my publisher was aghast at my referring to smokers as "dumb," because "no potential reader of this book," he insisted, "could possibly be dumb"—a view no doubt partially due to his concern that if I kept referring to smokers as dumb no smoker would buy this book, thus shutting out a potential market of several million people. But hey, I calls them as I sees them.

So as I said, I didn't want to do this chapter. I must say, however, that once I started to write it, I felt I had to give it my best shot, in part because my publisher also played the old guilt card.

"Just think," he said to me on that freezing morning in May (we live in Vancouver, after all) when I told him I'd omitted this chapter from the book, "about all the good you would be doing, Art, if only a few young persons reading this were moved to question why they're still smoking."

"Just think of all the young people you could help, Art," he repeated as he toted up figures on his calculator, "you who are so good at talking to young people," at which point I am sure I saw some of the butter that had melted in his mouth dribble onto his chin.

So, despite my reservations (what young person would ever be caught reading any book about health, I ask you?), I gave in because even if there is only an infinitesimally small chance my publisher is right, even if only one young person out there, who discovers his teacher's copy of this book open at this chapter while waiting for his detention, or one smoking adult, who reads his doctor's copy of this book while recovering in the OR after his colonoscopy, subsequently decides to quit smoking as a result of what he read here, it will indeed be worth all this effort.

And it's not that big a stretch, I suppose, given that statistics tell us that, in overwhelming numbers, smokers want to quit smoking. Indeed, most smokers regret ever having taken up the habit in the first place, and a vast majority claim they would give up smoking, if only, if only...

Why People Smoke

So why does anyone with a measurable IQ start to smoke in the first place, and even more to the point, why does any smoker continue smoking, especially given the fact that they're paying for the privilege of killing themselves slowly?

The major reason is clearly that smoking is highly addictive. A study that got a lot of publicity concluded that it took an average of only three weeks—three weeks!—for a teenage girl to get hooked on smoking after puffing on her first cigarette, even if she was only smoking "occasionally" (defined as "as little as two cigarettes a day, one day a week") to start. It took boys somewhat longer (boys *are* slower, after all), but it still took only six months for teenage males to get firmly hooked after first beginning to smoke. According to the head researcher, "some... kids [get] hooked within a few days of starting to smoke," which is scary news indeed.

And of course, it's not just young people who are addicted to smoking. According to one survey from Europe, over 60 percent of smokers in the U.K., Spain, France, and Sweden would rather give up sex for a month than put their cigarettes away for a similar length of time, which either confirms the fact that smoking is bloody hard to give up or tells you that sex in Europe isn't quite what most of us imagine it to be.

An American study found that over 25 percent of smokers who'd been diagnosed with a head and neck cancer were not able to quit smoking, even though they knew that continuing to smoke would severely affect their ability to survive or even to live a normal life in the little time they had left—head and neck cancers often cause a great deal of difficulty in swallowing, sipping fluids, talking, and even breathing.

Part of the reason smoking is so hard to quit is that nicotine has been shown to stimulate centers in the brain that are often associated with other forms of intense pleasure, such as watching Germany lose a soccer match or seeing Toronto get kicked out of the hockey playoffs—again.

Another reason so many people smoke is that it's seen to be sexy. There is a substantial subset of smokers (especially young ones, and alas, especially young women) who think that it's cool to be seen with a lit tube of dried leaf. This is not helped by the fact that Hollywood movies show us characters waving cigarettes around as if the latter were magic wands. Invariably, those smoking movie characters are beautiful or handsome and charming, like Julia Roberts, though in real life, smokers are mostly lined, decrepit, smelly, foul-breathed geezers with whom you would be reluctant to exchange pleasantries, let alone bodily fluids.

Some people, especially young girls, also smoke because they think it helps them control their weight. At a wedding dinner once I sat next to the girlfriend of one of my son's friends, who ate nothing but two let-tuce leaves—small ones they were, too—and who left to smoke (or throw up the lettuce) on several occasions. She looked thinner than her dinner, by the way.

But she was only doing what so many other young women do. In a re-cent American survey that spanned several years, one in four girls even-tually started smoking, and those young girls who most wanted to be thin on initial interviewing were much more likely to end up smoking down the road than girls who were not as concerned about their weight.

Health Risks of Smoking

Basically, smoking destroys everything between your brain and your balls.

I'm going to highlight that, just so you can easily recall it at night in bed when you have time to ponder some of life's deeper questions: *smoking batters your brains to your balls*, or, as the intellectuals out there might prefer, *smoking smashes your cerebrum to your sex.*

For those readers without balls, not to worry, because smoking makes an omelet of your eggs instead.

How bad is it to smoke? Worse than you think. Smoking is the lead-ing cause of premature death in the Western world and reduces average life expectancy by anywhere from eight to 25 years. According to some charts calculating risk of death that were published in the *Journal of the National Cancer Institute,* whereas a nonsmoking 60-year-old male has about a 15 percent chance of dying over the next decade, his smoking brother's risk is nearly 35 percent. For 60-year-old women, the risk of dying over the next decade doubles in smokers from about 10 percent to about 20 percent. That's because smoke and tar contain at least 4,000 known chemicals, including such yummy stuff as cyanide, ben-zene, ammonia, and carbon monoxide, none of which could possibly do you any good and all of which cause you much harm.

AGING

Nicotine and its byproducts speed the rate at which your tissues age. In other words, the more you smoke, the sooner you're a geezer. And this holds for all your tissues, not just the visible ones. In the Harvard Study of Adult Development, the single strongest predictor of "healthy physical aging" was "not being a smoker" (or having stopped smoking by one's mid-forties).

SKIN AND HAIR

If you're a smoker who can't afford Botox, by the time you hit late middle age you will often look many years older than your chronological age. To a twenty-something coolly exhaling a big gray cloud of smoke, I would say: "You know what Bob Dylan and Keith Richards look like? (Yes, they're still alive.) Well, that's what you're going to look like in a few years, too, baby. Want a light?"

Smoking not only causes wrinkles but also causes them to be deeper on average than regular age-related wrinkles, because smoking helps kill the collagen content of the skin, that stuff that makes your skin elastic. Collagen deteriorates naturally with time, anyway, and if you want to see that in action, just pinch yourself on the top of your hands one day when you see a beautiful young server approach your table to get your bar order. Then pinch her on her hand when she gets there, and as the bouncers are throwing you out, be sure to notice how quickly her skin returns to its resting state while yours is probably still taking its time to settle down. That's what happens when collagen deteriorates.

But collagen deteriorates much faster in smokers. Collagen in the skin also deteriorates much faster with exposure to sunlight, so there's really no mystery as to why people who smoke and lie in the sun a lot end up looking as if they should be skinned and their hides hung over the mantel. And here's an added bonus, smokers, if you're after that premature mature look: smoking also increases the amount of gray hair you have — if, that is, you still have hair, because smoking also raises the risk of premature baldness.

Now, on to the insides.

BRAIN

Let's start at the top (in some smokers, this is actually closer to the bottom, but hey, enough "dumb" references for now). What happens to brains exposed to continuous streams of nicotine and 4,000 other toxic products? They deteriorate; they fail; they become kaput. In other words, their owners become no-brainers. A study cited in the *American Journal of Epidemiology* on a bunch of smokers from the Netherlands (where the dikes are strong, and so are the men) found that smokers scored significantly lower than nonsmokers on tests of "mental speed" and "flexibility."

In fact, the smokers scored lower by quite a substantial margin—the researchers estimate that smokers seemed to be about "four years older" in mental speed and flexibility at a time of life when "older" is not better. Another recent study found that smokers who continue to puff away through middle age have significantly poorer memories than smokers who quit before their forties.

Several studies also conclude that smokers have significantly higher risks of developing Alzheimer's disease and other forms of dementia than nonsmokers. One study from Sweden found that the risk of Alzheimer's disease was double in smokers compared with nonsmokers.

But wait, there's more. As elderly smokers who have somehow managed to make it to old age with most of their brain function intact live on, they also have "more rapid decline in mental faculties," such as those involved in new learning and judgment, than do nonsmoking seniors—which may explain the delusions of the old army vet I mentioned earlier.

Smoking also affects brain function by raising the risk of stroke by anywhere from two to three times. According to one recent study, the risk of hemorrhagic stroke goes up in direct proportion to the number of cigarettes smoked over a lifetime. Researchers also speculate that smoking leads to multiple small strokes (in both the gray and white matter) that impair mental functioning (and possibly raise the risk of dementia) without necessarily producing any early, readily recognizable symptoms.

MOOD AND PERSONALITY

Many smokers argue that one of the main reasons they continue smoking is that it helps them stay calm. Surveys reveal that smokers do rely on cigarettes to deal with mood alterations, and according to at least one small study from California, the expectations of what smoking can do for anxiety and mood differ between the sexes. Male smokers are more likely to light up when they need to "wake themselves up," such as when they're accompanying their wives to a dinner party, perhaps, or to buy new drapes (by the way, I refer to that period when a wife, to the amazement of her clueless husband, decides to replace the drapes—or blinds or paint or carpets or bathrooms—as "renopause," and I'm trying to interest drug companies in developing a hormonal treatment for it). Male smokers also tend to light up when they're angry, which makes sense, I suppose, because now that we no longer have swords to pull out to indicate our rage a-building, men need some other phallic thingie to wave at the object of their anger. Women, in contrast, tend to smoke when they're happy, even euphoric, such as when they find out that they spent $5 less on a pair of shoes than their sister did.

As for the notion that smoking has a calming effect, there's lots of evidence that smoking may actually raise anxiety levels. A study of 700 adolescents who were followed into early adulthood concluded that problems such as panic attacks and generalized anxiety were much more common among heavy smokers than nonsmokers, not because the smokers were predestined to be anxious and to panic but rather because smoking aggravates both those emotional states. So, rather than decreasing anxiety—through a nicotine effect on the brain— smoking may actually raise the level of anxiety in some vulnerable individuals.

EYES

Smokers are more at risk of age-related maculopathy, the leading cause of blindness in North America, as well as cataracts.

EARS

Smokers have much faster and more significant deterioration in hearing than do nonsmokers. I'll repeat that in a louder voice: SMOKING DESTROYS YOUR HEARING. You're welcome.

NOSE AND MOUTH

Smoking destroys the senses of taste and smell and raises the risk of inflammation of the nose, throat, and sinuses (rhinitis and sinusitis).

Smoking is also a major cause of gingivitis, periodontal disease, and dental caries, also known as rotten gums and rotting teeth.

RESPIRATORY SYSTEM

Smokers have much higher rates of all sorts of chronic respiratory problems, including the big three: emphysema, chronic bronchitis, and asthma. They also have a much higher risk of acute respiratory infections, such as pneumonia and acute bronchitis, in part because smoking dulls the coughing reflex, so smokers have lots of trouble coughing up all that gunk they produce.

CARDIOVASCULAR SYSTEM

According to the British Heart Foundation, at least one-fifth of all heart attack deaths in men—and remember that heart attacks are by far the leading cause of death in men in the developed world, and yes, that includes Scotland—are directly attributable to smoking, making it the number one cause of premature death. Another study concluded that men who smoke have a 50 percent greater risk of dying from a heart attack than do nonsmoking men.

And women? Just as bad, of course. Smoking women have an 80 percent greater risk of heart attack than do their nonsmoking sisters, and the truly horrid thing is that far too many women smokers don't seem to know about their increased risk of heart disease. For one thing, they don't want to know, and for another, because women took up smoking in large numbers considerably later than men did, they have begun to suffer the deleterious effects relatively recently. As a result, many women still do not link their smoking to potential heart problems.

And it doesn't take much smoking to get a lethal effect. According to a great Danish study, smoking as few as three to five cigarettes a day doubles the risk of heart attack for women. For men, the risk is doubled with six to nine daily coffin nails, a level that is generally viewed to be a "light" smoking habit.

And for those Clinton wannabes who think they're fooling the Grim Reaper (or the special prosecutor) by not inhaling, you're not really fooling anyone, because in this study, the risk of heart attack was

doubled even in those who didn't inhale the toxic fumes their cigarettes produced.

So how does smoking do all that damage to the cardiovascular system? In many ways. Smoking:

- Alters lipid levels, leading to lower HDL and higher LDL levels.
- Harms blood vessels directly.
- Thickens the blood, leading to a higher risk of clots.
- Raises blood pressure.
- Increases the direct damage caused to heart cells from free radicals.
- Has an immediate effect on the sympathetic nervous system, raising
  blood pressure, for example, in the short term.
- Worsens the negative consequences of chronic inflammation.

People with chronic infections such as gingivitis or ulcers are already
known to be at significantly raised risk of heart attack and stroke (see
chapter 1), but according to an Italian study, if such people are exposed
to smoke, either because they themselves smoke or because they are
forced to inhale passive smoke, they are much more likely to experience accelerated atherosclerosis than are people who have early heart
disease but who don't smoke or inhale passive smoke. These Italian researchers claim that this effect on a smoker's health persists for up to 10
years after the smoker has quit his nasty habit.

This finding may also help explain why not every smoker develops
heart disease. There may be some subgroups of smokers, such as those
who have chronic infections, who are much more at risk from the toxic
effects of smoke than are other smokers, though that is certainly not to
say that if you don't have evidence of a chronic infection you can safely
light up.

Smoking also:

- Significantly raises the risk of peripheral artery disease, that terrible
  disability that often results in major pain in the limbs with any
  effort, including, in the worst cases, just taking a few steps.
- Increases the chances of developing those less-than-beautiful vari-
  cose veins that are every woman's nightmare.

- Increases the risk of developing aneurysms, which are weakenings in blood vessels that have the nasty tendency to rupture and kill many people every year.

All in all, then, it's no surprise that according to some studies and according to most experts, giving up smoking does at least as much good in reducing one's risk of heart attack as does taking the most effective cardio-protective medications.

STOMACH AND GUT
Smoking has long been listed as a risk factor for ulcers (though a few recent studies have thrown some doubt on that association). Smoking has also been shown to impair reflexes in the throat and esophagus that keep digestive acids down in the stomach where they are supposed to stay, thus raising the risk of gastro-esophageal reflux disease, or GERD. Down in the colon, smoking raises the risk of diverticulitis, which is a condition in which the bowel develops out-pouchings that become inflamed and often infected.

KIDNEY DISEASE AND BLADDER
Male smokers are over three times as likely to end up with impaired kidney function as are their nonsmoking brothers. Both men and women smokers with high blood pressure and/or diabetes end up with more kidney failure than do nonsmoking hypertensives and diabetics. And women smokers are also more likely to end up incontinent.

MALE GENITOURINARY SYSTEM
Smoking balls up a man's love life, so guys, if you want to be a lover or a father or both, stop smoking. Not only will you be better able to attract women when you stop smelling of cigarette fumes and when your breath stops reeking, but if you continue smoking, you also impair your ability to, you know, do it, and even more, to do it successfully.

Smoking is a major cause of erectile dysfunction, or ED, that problem that used to be known more accurately as impotence. In a recent review from China, middle-aged men who smoked had a 60 percent higher risk of ED than did nonsmokers. Smoking also reduces sperm density (sperm are like men: much more valuable when they're dense), reduces sperm motility, and leads to oxidative damage in sperm, which may be enough to tip the scales and move a borderline fertile man into the frustrating world of being relatively infertile.

FEMALE REPRODUCTIVE SYSTEM
In women, smoking raises the risks of:

- Infertility
- Ectopic pregnancy

A pregnant woman who smokes has a much higher risk of suffering pregnancy-related and labor-connected complications. Also, her baby has a higher risk of:

- Being stillborn.
- Having a low birth weight.
- Being premature.
- Having birth defects (in part because smoking also reduces the levels of folic acid in the blood, a vitamin known to reduce the risk of several birth defects).
- Having genetic and chromosomal abnormalities.
- Dying during the postpartum period.
- Dying of SIDS (smoking is the most easily controlled risk factor for SIDS, or sudden infant death syndrome).
- Being obese. According to German researchers, women who smoke while pregnant raise the chances of that particular child becoming obese as he grows. Their conclusion was that maternal smoking is as bad for a kid's eventual waistline as is frequent television viewing and regular playing of video games (such as those popular German video games "Move the Trains on Time" and "Suck Up to France").

Women who smoke are also more likely to suffer:

- Earlier menopause. Although that may at first sound like a good thing (no periods, no pads, no PMS), it's not really, since early

menopause is also tied to future health rates such as higher risks of heart disease and osteoporosis.
- More hot flashes, and more severe hot flashes, during menopause.

CANCERS

Smoking directly causes approximately 30 percent of cancer deaths and is clearly the single most controllable risk factor for cancer. Smokers who get cancer are also much more likely to be diagnosed with advanced and untreatable cancers than are nonsmokers.

Cancers that are either caused by or aggravated by smoking include:

- Lung cancer. Lung cancer is the leading cause of cancer death in the United States and Canada. Male smokers are 22 to 23 times as likely to die from lung cancer and women smokers are 12 to 13 times as likely to die from lung cancer than nonsmokers. Lest you dismiss that with a shrug, thinking that cancer only kills old folks, let me tell you that in Canada, 40 percent of lung cancer deaths occur in people under the age of 65.
- Oral cancer: nasal cavities, sinuses, mouth, pharynx, throat, larynx.
- Esophageal cancer.
- Stomach cancer.
- Pancreatic cancer. One recent study concluded that if all the smokers in the EU were to quit smoking, the number of cases of pancreatic cancer would drop by 150,000 in Europe by 2010.
- Cervical cancer. Women who are already infected with the human papilloma virus, or HPV, the main cause of cervical cancer, have a much higher rate of developing frank cervical cancer if they also smoke. What makes this connection particularly troubling is that the rate of HPV infection is rising quickly in young women (largely because HPV infection rarely produces symptoms), and since HPV is currently incurable (like your kids, it's with you for life), we may eventually see a dramatic spike in cervical cancer cases in many of those young women smokers.
- Colon cancer. Smoking has been strongly linked to a rise in the risk of colorectal polyps, which, if untreated, can go on to become colon cancer, so smoking hits you in the arse, as well.

- Liver cancer.
- Kidney cancer.
- Bladder cancer.
- Ureter cancer.
- Prostate cancer. Younger men who smoke are more likely to be diagnosed with advanced prostate cancer than are nonsmoking young men.
- Uterine cancer.
- Skin cancer.
- Bone marrow cancer.
- Leukemia.
- Lymphoma. Smoking not only can cause cancers of the lymph gland system, such as Hodgkin's disease and others, but according to one study, can also transform manageable lymph gland malignancies into more lethal types.
- Breast cancer. A recent study in the *American Journal of Epidemiology* concluded that the risk of breast cancer goes up directly with the amount smoked; the longer a woman has smoked and the more cigarettes she has consumed, the higher her eventual risk of breast cancer. The longer she has stopped smoking, however, the lower her risk becomes. This study also found that women exposed to significant amounts of passive smoke are also at greater risk of breast cancer.

◆ ———————————————————————— ◆

YOUNG GIRLS, SMOKING, AND BREAST CANCER

A Canadian study found that girls who begin to smoke during their early teenage years, that is, within five years of commencing menstruation, have up to a 70 percent higher risk of breast cancer later in life than do girls who either don't smoke or postpone their first cigarettes until they're much older, perhaps because breast tissue in those early postmenarche years is still immature and forming, and any toxic effect of smoking is multiplied on that very active, young tissue. Some authorities want to highlight these findings to young women, on the assumption that the fear of breast cancer down the line may deter some of them from smoking. Young girls, after all, are the demographic group in whom smoking rates are rising most rapidly. I'm all for informing young people of risks, but as a lifelong cynic who worked for many years in a free clinic that catered to adolescents and young adults, I doubt that an ad campaign that trumpets these findings is going to persuade any young girl to either postpone or quit smoking. To a young girl, anything that's going to happen 30, 20, 10, or even one year down the line is like, you know, so last week.

◆ ──────────────────────────────── ◆

BONES, JOINTS, AND MUSCLES

Smoking is a major risk factor for the bone-thinning disease of osteo-porosis, and postmenopausal women who smoke are much more likely than their nonsmoking sisters to fracture a hip. As for joints (the kind you injure, not the kind you inhale), a survey of 54,000 Puerto Ricans found that arthritis is more common in people who have smoked at any point, so even if you've only smoked when you were a teenage dummy, your eventual risk of arthritis is still higher than that of your self-righteous wife who's never lit up in her life.

PAIN

A survey from Britain found that smokers complained of more "dis-comforting or disabling musculo-skeletal pain" than nonsmokers, stuff like pain in the shoulders, hands, and knees and especially in the back—the kind of pain you get, in other words, after you've moved the couch for the eighth time because the room still doesn't look right. Or so says my wife, whenever I try to get her to move ours.

And please note, the musculo-skeletal pain these people were expe-riencing was not some minor problem, but rather the kind of pain that prevented many of them from going to work or doing housework. (But as a househusband, I wonder, is that always a bad thing?)

Smokers are much more likely to report feeling discomforting pain than are nonsmokers because:

• Nicotine damages tissues so that they are more easily inflamed with a smaller amount of irritation than are the tissues of nonsmokers.

- Smoking affects blood vessels so that the chemicals that dampen pain may simply not get to the inflamed areas as easily.
- Nicotine damages either the brain or neurological tissue (or both) so that smokers feel pain much more readily than do nonsmokers, that is, at lower levels of injury.
- Smokers may simply be the kind of people who are predisposed to feeling pain at lower levels than nonsmokers even before they take up their suicidal habit.

MORE GENERAL PROBLEMS

- Smokers are three times as likely as nonsmokers to get diabetes, and once they do get it, smokers have a tougher time controlling their blood sugar levels than do nonsmoking diabetics.
- Some studies have found increased risks of thyroid disease in smokers, though others have not. No study has ever found, however, that smoking is good for your thyroid.
- Smoking also leads to vitamin abnormalities such as low blood levels of the carotenoids, vitamin B12, vitamin C, and perhaps most important, vitamin D, which may partly explain why smokers are so much more prone to cancers and other diseases that involve damage to DNA.

BENEFITS OF QUITTING

If smoking is so bad for you, do we have any proof that quitting smoking reverses any of the damage that a long history of smoking has already produced? The simple answer (as Sally told Harry) is "Yes, yes, yes, yes, yes, yes, yes" (my wife came up with that way before Meg Ryan, by the way, that day back in 1977 when I suggested we take separate vacations).

A huge 16-year study for the Agency of Health Care Policy and Research in the U.S. determined that people who stop smoking lower their risks of smoking-related disease so much that they are eventually no more likely to be hospitalized for a smoking-related disorder than is someone who's never smoked at all. If they don't quit, however, men who smoke are 33 percent more likely to end up in hospital than their nonsmoking brothers.

Although it's not quite as bad for women smokers, they're still significantly more likely to end up in the hospital than are their nonsmoking sisters.

The benefits of quitting kick in pretty quickly, too. Within one year of quitting smoking, the risks of suffering a heart attack drop significantly, and after 10 years, the risk is down to that of a lifelong nonsmoker. The risks of lung and other cancers, as well as the risk of dying from any cause, also drop dramatically after 15 years or more of not smoking. However, those risks always remain somewhat higher than those of a lifelong nonsmoker.

So that's what's in it for anyone who quits. And if you're a parent, there's one other major benefit: the best protection you can offer your children against becoming smokers themselves is to give up your habit, since smoking parents tend to have kids who also end up smoking. One intriguing study concluded that Latino boys who "were asked to light cigarettes for their parents were the most likely to become teenage smokers." Doh!

And for those parents who take the attitude that "Well, I plan to quit for Junior's sake, but I think I'll wait till he's 30," you really should feel more of an urgency about quitting. A recent study published in the journal *Addiction* found that a smoking parent most reduces the risk that his children will be smokers if the parent quits his habit before the kid hits the age of eight or nine. After that, the parent's quitting has much less effect on the child's risk of smoking.

◆ ────────────────────────────────── ◆

HOW TO QUIT SMOKING

A study published in the journal *Pediatrics* underlines just how hard it is to give up smoking. Researchers took aside the parents of kids who'd been admitted to hospital with a severe respiratory problem, which is nearly always caused or at the very least significantly aggravated by a parent's smoking, and gave them intense stop-smoking therapy consisting of "the works": written material, free nicotine replacement therapy, telephone counseling, and doctor referrals. About the only thing these researchers didn't do for these parents was to go over to the smokers' houses to blow the matches out when they lit up. What's more, the smokers were offered these therapies in a "nonthreatening, motivational," guilt-free manner, another stop-smoking tactic intended to get the best possible results from attempts to quit. Yet even with all these intense efforts, less than half of the parents even tried to quit, most of the quitters lasted less than 24 hours, and only about 20 percent of them reported being off smokes after two months (the real number was likely lower, because at least a few of them probably lied to the researchers). So I acknowledge that it's very hard to quit.

That said, studies find that 50 percent of smokers do eventually quit, so it's always worth a try.

How do you do it? Well, as with the guy who built the Panama Canal, it's best to start with a plan. Among the things to consider are the following:

- Number one with a bullet: find out as much about smoking and how to quit as you can (some of which you are clearly doing, of course, by reading this chapter). I also suggest visiting some of the excellent Web sites dedicated to letting you know about all your stop-smoking options, such as those programs run by the various lung and chest associations.
- If you decide you need professional help, my strong advice is to pay for some direct counseling and not to rely primarily on your poorly paid, time-challenged family doc (however, those family doctors who do take a special interest in helping patients quit smoking undoubtedly achieve excellent results.)
- Number three, but also with a bullet: make some other lifestyle changes, such as working out more and eating more healthfully. But why should you make such changes while battling your addiction? First, when you are as determined as you are at this moment to do so much for yourself, it's a great opportunity to make those other health adjustments that you ought to make, anyway—start afresh, in other words. Second, although I don't have the science to back me up, I firmly believe that all those other efforts to live more healthfully make it easier to achieve your goal of living without smoke in your life. Third, better lifestyle habits also help your body recover from the awful things you've already done to it by all that smoking. For example, a study from Ireland found that smokers could help speed up the repair to the damage in their arteries caused by smoking if they lustily sang "Carrickfergus" twice an evening at the pub. (Just joking.) The real conclusion was that a diet

high in fish oils repaired smokers' arteries. As you no doubt recall from chapter 3, fish oils can help arteries stay flexible, and fish oils may be so powerful that they can even repair the arteries of smokers. Finally, yes, you are likely to gain a few pounds when you quit smoking, so if you start running or start eating better, that weight gain will be held to a minimum.

- If your spouse smokes, get him or her to quit smoking, too. Several studies have determined that in a two-smoker household, it's far easier for a smoker to be successful at quitting smoking if his or her spouse makes an attempt to stop at the same time.

- Make a determination to quit entirely. I simply can't believe in those fairyland schedules and plans in which you cut down the number of cigarettes you smoke per day or switch to lighter brands, or even, as some in the cancer-promoting smoking industry would now have you do, switch to "safer nicotine-reduced cigarettes" or other nicotine-containing products, such as nicotine-laced lollipops. Unfortunately, this "safer cigarette" bandwagon is even gathering lots of somber scientists aboard, who seem to have become convinced that there are some hard-core smokers out there (no doubt determined by everyone's fall-back scapegoat of genetic susceptibility) who cannot quit no matter what help they receive, so let's at least try to minimize the damage they do themselves, by giving them an easier out than all-or-none quitting.

To me, though, anything short of quitting completely is like saying that you're going to stop beating your children one day by hitting them fewer times a week or that you will minimize the hurt you cause them by switching your strap for a duster. There's ample evidence that even as few as three cigarettes a day lead to much higher risks of many diseases. One study that looked at the effect that smoking has on blood vessels concluded that there was no difference between the blood vessels of people who smoked three cigarettes a day and those who smoked 20 a day.

Another study on the effects of cutting down smoking found no difference in the risks of being admitted to hospital with a flare-up of chronic obstructive pulmonary disease, or COPD, between people who smoked more than 15 cigarettes a day and those who continued to puff away at half that number; of course, those who quit entirely markedly reduced their chances of going to hospital with a COPD flare-up.

So, smokers, if you want to quit, heed the words of women all over the world: be hard or don't bother—it really is all or nothing.

- Make a list of the times and places you smoke the most. Then you can try to avoid these cues or at the very least minimize the role they play in your smoking life.
- Pick a specific date and tell everyone you know that you're going to quit on that day. Pile the pressure on yourself, because those others—your friends, your colleagues, your spouse, and best of all, your judgmental and unsparing kids—may help you stick with the program when you're in danger of slipping up.
- Finally, pick a stop-smoking method.

COLD TURKEY

Cold turkey is every smoker's favorite stop-smoking method. Most smokers like cold turkey so much, in fact, that they've used it at least a dozen times.

Why are smokers so enamored of cold turkey? Because you can do it anytime you want with absolutely no cost and without any telltale signs to let others know that's what you're doing. Only thing is, most smokers can't do it.

Thus, compared with all other stop-smoking methods, cold turkey has the lowest rate of abstention (that means the fewest people still not smoking) at one year (about 4 to 6 percent). One important reason for this seemingly low success rate is that cold turkey tends to attract a great many not completely serious candidates. So although it's hard to judge how effective this method is in people who really, really, really want to quit, it's probably way better than 4 percent. Which is why I'd encourage anyone who wants to quit to do it on any day they choose to start, without waiting for the stars to be more propitious.

COUNSELING

Most doctors don't take a strong enough interest in helping their patients quit smoking, in large part because (1) doctors don't feel it's worth the effort to help a smoker quit, since most smokers are bound to fail in any individual attempt to quit, and (2) doctors usually don't get paid for stop-smoking counseling. But if your doctor is willing to spend the time and effort to help you quit, studies show that you have a much greater chance of succeeding with her help. So, sidle over to your doctor's office, and see if she's able and willing to spend the time with you. If she is, go for it.

If she's not, then find yourself a counselor to help you through the hard first few weeks, cost permitting. Also, if you can find a support group such as Nicotine Anonymous, join it, time and your personality permitting.

NICOTINE REPLACEMENT

Nicotine replacement therapy (NR) is more effective than cold turkey; according to most studies, anywhere from 14 to 20 percent of people on NR are cigarette-free at one year, and that rate goes up if NR is combined with other stop-smoking methods. That said, recent data have revealed that NR therapy may not be as effective as was originally hyped, which would make it no different from any other recent "miracle" intervention (see hormone replacement therapy for menopause, Fen-Phen for weight reduction, Viagra for, well, you know). According to a study in the *Journal of the American Medical Association*, which was in turn based on several large surveys done among California smokers, nicotine replacement therapies, which became widely available in 1996, had no measurable effect on the ability of heavy smokers (over 15 cigarettes a day) to stay off cigarettes in the long term. In other words, long-term successful smoking cessation was no higher in the years after nicotine replacement became available than it had been in the years before, though there is some evidence that heavy smokers may try to quit more often with the help of NR. These researchers also concluded that there was insufficient evidence to indicate that light smokers could be helped to quit either in the short term or the long term with NR, which is considerably more pessimistic than the conclusions drawn from most other studies.

Four forms of NR therapy are on the market: gum, skin patch, nasal spray, and inhaler (though you can bet there will eventually be several other forms available, including, I'm sure, an injectable device to deliver nicotine directly to the bloodstream if not directly to the brain), and each has been found to be effective at helping some smokers quit.

But how do they stack up against each other? An American study published in the *Archives of Internal Medicine* tried to come up with an answer, and the results were interesting. The only form of NR in which compliance was judged to be adequate (in other words, the only method that real people in the real world stuck to in any significant numbers) was the patch (why people couldn't stick with gum is something I really don't get, but hey, these are smokers, after all).

Unsurprisingly, the nasal spray was cited as having the most troublesome side effects, and the inhaler was deemed to be the most "embarrassing" to use. (So let me see if I have this right: it's not embarrassing to put a cigarette in your mouth and to drip ashes all over the front porch, but hey, it *is* embarrassing to put an inhaler in your mouth for 10 seconds to indicate that you're trying to get off cigarettes. I just don't understand smokers.)

When it came to the most important aspects of how well they worked in getting smokers to quit, all four NR therapies were fairly equivalent in helping with withdrawal symptoms, in helping a smoker deal with the mental aspects of trying not to smoke, and in helping control weight gain up to 12 weeks. One important difference, though, was that at 12 weeks post-quitting, the least-liked method, the nasal spray, was the most effective at having kept smokers off their cigarettes for those three months, perhaps because it delivers the fastest jolt of nicotine.

But the bottom line is that for someone who is committed to quitting, all the forms of NR are probably pretty much equivalent, a conclusion drawn by another study that compared over-the-counter NR therapies with prescription forms of the same. At both six weeks and six months, it doesn't really matter which form of NR you choose—your chances of success are pretty much the same. In this study at least, over-the-counter nicotine gum had a bit of a better record than prescription patches, mostly because, the researchers speculate, patients who choose gum are usually fairly strongly self-motivated, whereas doctors have a lot to do with the success of patches, and most doctors simply do not spend the time or effort to reinforce the need to stick with the patches.

In summary, then:

- First, choose the NR method you think you may stick with. I mean, if you hate putting anything in your nose, then don't pick the nasal spray, and if you have trouble chewing gum and doing something else at the same time, then don't choose gum.

- Second, try to buttress your NR method with some added therapy, such as Zyban (see below), or counseling that costs you tons of money, because the more you pay for a therapy, the more likely it is that you're going to work hard at it. (Which is, after all, the real secret behind the success of so many "saved" marriages: the couples paid for the counseling, and damned if they're going to admit that it was a waste of money and effort, so why not stick it out, eh? At least that's what my wife keeps saying, so please don't tell her that I never paid the therapist.)

Side effects of NR include the usual suspects:

- Headaches
- Nausea
- Stomach upsets

One of the more troublesome early problems, especially in those who start on higher doses, is sleep disturbance, but thankfully, it is usually transient.

Problems peculiar to nicotine gum include the fact that it has to be chewed slowly and that some substances that you might also want to indulge in at the same time (coffee, for example, or soft drinks) might interfere with its efficacy.

Finally, here are a couple of cautions about nicotine replacement therapy:

- First, never smoke while you're on NR, because your nicotine level may shoot up too high.
- Lots of people stay on NR therapies for way too long. I mean, after a month or so, or at most two months, you should definitely have lowered your nicotine dose significantly, and if you haven't, then you've got to wonder if this is what you want to be doing.

"But why not simply continue with nicotine replacement forever?" some of you may ask. Two reasons. First, I'm convinced that NR creates its own dependency—not perhaps a chemical or physiological dependency, meaning that you don't really get wired to patches and nasal sprays, but rather a psychological dependency, an intense feeling that you can't really get away from the nicotine replacement without jeopardizing the previous month-long (or, more often, months-long) effort. But hey, as any six-year-old can tell you, if you really want to ride that bike, you've got to throw the training wheels away sooner or later, and with nicotine replacement, the sooner, the better.

Also, although we've always believed that it's the tar in cigarettes that causes most of the damage, especially smoking-related cancers, according to several small studies it may be nicotine itself that is carcinogenic. Studies have shown that nicotine may promote "cancer development and progression" and that nicotine alone may also narrow arteries, which would be true for any form of nicotine that got into you. In other words, as I said earlier, you want to get off nicotine sooner rather than later.

DRUGS

Zyban
Zyban (or Wellbutrin) is the cure-de-jour for smoking cessation, and indeed, the evidence in its favor is impressive. Some studies have found that twice as many smokers were able to quit smoking if they were taking Zyban than if they were taking a placebo.

Zyban is also very useful in buttressing nicotine replacement therapy, so the combination of NR and Zyban seems to work better than either method alone. Although Zyban works well in every demographic group, according to one study, it may be most effective in older males and those who smoke fewer than 30 cigarettes a day.

Zyban is pretty well tolerated in general. The most common side effects, which, happily are usually temporary and mild, include:

- Nausea
- Headaches
- Shakiness

The more troublesome common side effects are:

- Dry mouth
- Insomnia

The most worrying side effects are:

- Chest pain
- Palpitations
- Seizures

The estimated seizure rate in Zyban users is about 1 in 1,000, a rate that's much higher in people with a past history of seizure and those who are at high risk of seizure, which includes:

- Those with eating disorders, such as anorexia nervosa or bulimia.
- Those with a central nervous system tumor.
- Alcoholics.
- Those who are simultaneously withdrawing from alcohol or other drugs.
- People with a history of significant head trauma.
- Diabetics taking certain glucose-lowering medications.
- People on appetite-suppressing drugs.
- People on drugs that lower the threshold for seizure, such as some antidepressants.

For anyone at higher risk of seizure, the risks of taking Zyban must be very carefully balanced against the potential benefits.

Other drugs
Although Zyban is by far the favorite stop-smoking drug these days, other drugs have been used successfully to help smokers quit, including an older class of antidepressants (what did you think Zyban was, anyway?) called tricyclic antidepressants, such as nortriptyline. The problem is that these are not the easiest meds to take (they produce

troublesome side effects such as dry mouth and daytime fatigue, and on rare occasions they can cause dangerous cardiac complications), but they are much cheaper than Zyban and they might be worth a try, especially by people who may have taken them once before and are already familiar with the side effects.

One small study also found that the drug seligiline, used for the treatment of Parkinson's disease, may also be helpful in some smokers.

OTHER THERAPIES
This list is rather long and includes:

- Laser therapy
- Acupuncture
- Hypnosis
- Aversion therapy (in which, I presume, they show you pictures of smokers that turn your stomach, such as close-ups of Keith Richards)
- And many others

I'm afraid, however, that there are few objective studies to tell you how effective these are compared with placebo. But hey, if a placebo therapy works for you, then go for it. You have nothing to lose but your bucks. After all, some of my favorite drugs and therapies are placebos, only I never admit that to myself because then they'd stop working.

Research
"Is there anything else in that pipe, Art?" I can hear you asking with a silly grin on your face. Who says I'm the only one allowed to make awful jokes in this book?

Of course there is. Anything that would mimic the major effects that nicotine has on the brain should be an effective anti-smoking tool, and to that end, a recent study in the very focused journal *Nicotine and Tobacco Research* found that the drug bromocriptine, which mimics the action of the neurotransmitter dopamine and which has long been used to treat Parkinson's disease as well as some menstrual disorders, was also effective at lowering smokers' intake of cigarettes.

It's early days yet, as they say, and it's unlikely that smokers experience only one type of chemical "high" from their drug of choice. But if dopamine turns out to be a major player in smokers' need to keep puffing, you can bet that within a few years we will have much better dopamine simulators around, given the market there would be for such drugs.

Another study found a positive effect on smoking rates (that means the rates went down) from a drug called rimonabant, which is a "cannabinoid receptor agonist," meaning that it blocks the effect that cannabis has on the brain (so I suppose it prevents you getting ridiculously silly and eating too much, which I have been told occurs commonly in people who smoke pot).

But the real holy grail for smoking researchers is to come up with a vaccine that helps smokers kick their habit. To that end, a British company is working on a vaccine that "stops nicotine from entering the brain" (although I have to tell them that I already have such a device: it's called a nonsmoking wife).

Passive Smoke
Although this issue has not been entirely settled (some experts still argue that passive smoking is not harmful, but then some people also argue that the Taliban should never have been attacked), I am certain that passive smoking, formerly known as secondhand smoke (a name that lost out simply because, to people like my dad, "secondhand smoke" merely meant having a lit cigarette in each paw; he lived into his late eighties, by the way) does harm to anyone exposed to it. I thoroughly accept studies such as the one from the U.S. that concluded that passive smoking is the third leading cause of preventable death in the U.S., and one from the U.K. that concluded that passive smoking kills 900 office workers, 165 bar workers, and 145 manufacturing workers every year, or about three British workers every day of the year.

Fortunately, more and more governments are making it harder for insufferable smokers to light up and blow their toxins in an innocent's face. I mean, who would ever have predicted that even the Irish and Italians would one day pass laws banning smoking in restaurants and (Holy Mother of God) in pubs, too?

Governments are doing so because passive smoking couldn't possibly do anyone any good and it is very likely doing a lot of people a lot of harm. Furthermore, there is no known level of safe exposure, so even one inhalation of someone else's smoke is one inhalation too many. "Smokers' rights" is a concept as ridiculous as the idea of "women's rights" in Saudi Arabia.

Passive smoke has been linked to increased risks of:

- Heart disease
- Stroke
- Lung cancer
- Respiratory disorders
- Other malignancies, such as stomach cancer, liver cancer, kidney cancer, cervical cancer, and some types of leukemia
- Gum disease

But perhaps the most insidious effect of passive smoke is what it does to newborns and infants. Moms who smoke significantly raise the risk that their young babe might die of crib death, or sudden infant death syndrome (SIDS). Interestingly, according to at least one study done in rodents, nicotine by itself may raise the risk of SIDS because nicotine seems to have a dampening effect on receptors in the brain that are used to "wake us up" when oxygen levels get too low during sleep. This also raises the possibility that certain forms of nicotine replacement therapy that are heavily promoted for smoking cessation might also produce the same effect.

Infants growing up in a smoking environment also have higher rates of:

- Respiratory infections requiring hospitalization, such as bronchitis and pneumonia (even having a smoker go out of an infant's room to light up lowers that risk)
- Sore throats
- Sinusitis
- Ear infections
- Way more and way worse asthma
- Lung cancer, rare though those cancers may be in this age group

- Deficiencies in certain vitamins in their bloodstreams

Compared with the children of nonsmokers, the children of smokers are also more likely to have:

- Developmental defects
- Behavior problems
- ADHD (attention-deficit hyperactivity disorder)
- Social problems

And to top it all off, the children of smokers are much more likely to be smokers themselves.

You still want to light up another one, Dad?

Cigars and Pipes

I have to say a few words about cigars and pipes because as my cigar-chomping, poker-playing, beer-guzzling friend pointed out (I let her read this part of the manuscript), "All that stuff you wrote was about cigarettes, right?" Well, yes, the studies cited were done on cigarette smokers, but that's just because there are so many more of them (both cigarette smokers and studies about them). But despite the relative paucity of studies on cigar and pipe smokers, we still know that at the very least, cigar smoking is strongly related to a higher risk of several cancers—including oral, laryngeal, respiratory, and gastrointestinal cancers—and pipe smokers are at much higher risk of oral and lung cancers. As to the cardiovascular effects of smoking cigars or a pipe, let me ask you: when was the last time you saw a cigar smoker or pipe smoker run without quickly getting short of breath? Never mind, when was the last time you saw one even walk briskly?

Look, the bottom line is this: smoking is not good for you or any other living creature, no matter which form of smoke you choose to surround yourself with and no matter whether you inhale or not. Period.

Benefits of Nicotine

Finally, one of the world's shortest sections: the accumulated wisdom of Jean ("He is no moron, he is my friend") Chrétien. No, actually, it's this: the positive effects of nicotine.

Nicotine helps improve concentration, and perhaps short-term memory (ever meet a smoker who can't remember where his pack of smokes is?), and it may also have a slightly positive effect on the chances of developing Parkinson's disease. Thing is, smoking is much more likely to kill you before you have any chance to see if you get Parkinson's.

CHAPTER

8

Sleep

Some Snooze, They Lose; Some
Snooze, They Cruise

I don't mind going to bed on an empty stomach
as long as it's not mine.
MAE WEST

A FTER I DID the first seven chapters of this book, I naturally thought I was pretty close to the end. In fact, given that the manuscript was already one year overdue, I was certain that I was at the end. Imagine my surprise, then, when my editor called me after I submitted these chapters and said, "Hey!" (She and I are not very intimate.) "Hey! What about those chapters you owe me on sex and those other things that go with it?"

"Sex and those other things that go with it?" I can be as stupid as the next guy.

"Yes, it was in the proposal you sent me. Remember?"

Of course I didn't remember, since I had sent her that proposal so long ago. I'm a midlife man, after all, and I don't even remember what I said yesterday.

"Oh, yes," I bluffed. "Sex and those other things that go with it. Sure."

221

So I sat down and began to write some chapters about sex, drugs, and rock 'n' roll—until, that is, I got the bright idea that perhaps I should consult that outline first. Wouldn't you know it, two-thirds of sex, drugs, and rock 'n' roll were not in my original proposal.

Again, because I'm a midlifer, in my proposal, the chapters on sex and the things that go with it actually meant a discussion of sex, stress, and sleep. Well, what else does sex go with in middle age, eh?

So here is the first chapter on the three S's (in no order of importance—you have to decide that for yourself): sleep, stress, and (if you have the time and energy) sex.

Sleep is one of those things in life—sex, money, and fun are three others—that we only pay attention to when we don't have enough of them. And unfortunately it appears that we're getting less and less sleep than we used to. (I don't have the statistics for sex, money, and fun, but I imagine it's the same for them, too). In the U.S., a telephone survey found that over 60 percent of adults sleep only an average of seven hours a night, whereas a century ago, folks in North America were apparently averaging more than eight hours of sleep a night.

That's only an average, of course, so clearly some people get much less sleep than others. It's commonly believed that seniors are especially prone to not getting enough sleep, and indeed more than half the seniors questioned for a recent survey for the U.S. National Sleep Foundation claimed to be having trouble sleeping, though most also said they were getting about seven hours of sleep a night. Since that is in line with what the general adult population gets, perhaps seniors are not as badly off as they think—they may just like to complain. That said, sleep quality and sleep patterns do change with age: most seniors—men and women—do not sleep in on weekends, for example, which is why your mom always calls you at 7 AM on a Sunday and wonders why you're not up yet.

How Much Sleep Do You Need?

There are two important aspects to getting enough sleep: how long you sleep and what quality of sleep you get. A newborn requires 16 or more hours of sleep a day. By the end of primary school, that requirement goes down to about 10 hours. Although teenagers don't consider themselves kids, they are not yet adults, either, so most of them require nine or so hours of sleep a night to be fully rested the next day. For adults, it's commonly said they need an average of eight hours of sleep a night.

For example, recent findings from the Nurses' Health Study revealed that women who sleep *less or more* than an average of eight hours a night have a higher risk of heart disease (and diabetes) than women who sleep an average of eight hours a night. At one end of the spectrum, women who reported sleeping five or fewer hours a night had a 45 percent higher risk of heart disease (and a 30 percent greater risk of diabetes). At the other end, women who reported sleeping nine or more hours a night had a 38 percent greater risk of heart disease.

Before you settle on eight hours as the magic number to aim for, however, let me tell you that another study that followed over a million men and women for six years as part of the American Cancer Society's Cancer Prevention Study II (CPSII) found that those who slept seven hours a night on average had the best overall mortality. Those sleeping eight hours were 12 percent more likely to die within the six-year period than those sleeping seven hours, and even those who slept as little as five hours a night lived longer than those who needed eight hours or more. Just as interesting, suffering from occasional bouts of insomnia (doesn't everyone?) didn't affect individuals' life expectancies at all, except for this: people who took sleeping pills were more likely to die sooner than people who didn't take such drugs.

So is it seven or is it eight? The simple truth is that no one knows. Besides, there are plenty of seemingly normal people who do very well averaging much more and especially much less than that mid-range of seven to eight hours a night.

On the other side of the ledger, my wife sleeps an average of 12 hours a night. Well, to be fair, she says it's closer to nine, but I'm counting all those periods of time in the evening when she's clearly asleep, or at least not listening to me.

Adequate sleep also means getting enough good-quality sleep, including enough deep sleep and enough REM sleep. The bottom line, then, in determining how well you've slept is not just the number of hours you spent snoozing but rather how you feel the next day; if you feel sprightly and can function well, then you've probably had enough good-quality sleep the night before. But I must also stress that there is absolutely no proof that if you sleep more or less than seven to eight hours a night—and feel well rested the next day—you will do anything positive for your health by changing your sleep pattern.

What Does Sleep Do?

But what exactly does sleep do? No one knows for sure, but here are some of the things it seems to be necessary for:

- Proper growth and development.
- Energy conservation.
- Immune system functioning.
- Memory and cognitive functioning.
- Maybe even life itself. An intriguing theory that I am willing to buy has it that the reason women live longer than men is that women are better sleepers. Women sleep more soundly and are less put off by sleep disturbances than men, and these factors correlate with better immune functioning, better hormonal balance, and fewer signs of chronic inflammation. But these advantages are at least partially offset by the resulting lack of wisdom that comes to those of us who are awake to watch late-night TV shows.

Insomnia

The experts say that over 90 percent of people have trouble with sleep at least one time in their lives. I believe that the true figure is much closer to 100 percent since I don't know anyone who hasn't had at least an occasional problem falling asleep. But for most of us, problems with sleep are temporary and usually mitigated by a good home remedy, such as drinking a glass of warm milk or watching anything on the Parliamentary Channel or C-SPAN.

Insomnia can manifest itself as:

- Difficulty falling asleep.
- Frequent nighttime wakening.
- Difficulty falling back asleep after waking.
- Inadequate deep sleep.
- Unrefreshing sleep.
- Excessive daytime fatigue.

Temporary sleep disturbances may last up to a few weeks and are usually caused by:

- A specific stressful event, including the appearance of a new health condition.
- Poor sleep hygiene (see below).
- The use of certain medications such as bronchodilators, decongestants, diuretics, antidepressants (SSRI antidepressants such as Prozac are notorious for causing sleep problems), and antihistamines.
- Rebound insomnia (see below).
- Disruption of our internal 24-hour circadian rhythm clock, as with jet lag, for example.

For anywhere from 10 to 18 percent of the population, however, insomnia is a chronic problem, though difficulties with sleep usually don't occur every night.

There are many causes for chronic sleep disturbance, including:

- Psychological conditions, such as chronic anxiety, worrying about falling asleep, depression, or panic disorder.
- Chronic medical problems, including obesity, asthma, GERD, and many others.
- Pain.
- Sleep apnea (see below).
- Sleep disorders, such as periodic limb movement disorder.
- Substance abuse, including alcohol.
- Menopause and other hormonal conditions.
- Age. Sleep quality tends to deteriorate with age (more quickly in men than in women), but a lot of that has to do with the fact that chronic medical problems are much more common as we grow older. Even if a senior is disease-free, though, his sleep quality is still quite different than when he was younger—his sleep is lighter, he wakes more easily, he has more trouble falling back asleep, he has less REM sleep, and so on.

If you don't get enough sleep or enough good-quality sleep, you begin to build up a "sleep debt." Some experts believe that anyone who uses an alarm clock to wake up is sleep-deprived by definition and is building up a sleep debt. Building and owning a sleep debt is a very common problem, in part because it happens so quickly. In a recent study in the journal *Sleep*, researchers concluded that sleeping less than eight hours on average for as little as two weeks leads to a sleep debt equivalent to missing two full nights of sleep.

Most people don't realize that they are not functioning up to par because of a sleep debt, since the symptoms can be so subtle. I mean, how would most of us ever know that our memory was slightly poorer than normal since half of zero is still zero?

Given how important sleep is for normal functioning, it's no surprise that not getting enough sleep causes lots of problems:

- Subsequent daytime fatigue following even one night's poor or inadequate sleep.
- Lack of motivation. People who are often tired just don't try as hard as they would if they were rested (I excuse twenty-somethings from this claim, though, because they never try even when they're well rested). Just as bad, people who are sleep-deprived usually don't care that they're not trying as hard as they would if they were well rested.
- Poor performance. Surgeons, pilots, truckers, and others who don't get a good night's sleep perform more poorly on tests than when they do get enough sleep, information that may keep you up tonight if you're reading this before boarding a plane or before your prostate surgery. Just to keep you even more wakeful, one study found that the loss of one complete night's sleep (what happens to your usual medical intern, oh, about two nights a week, usually the night that you have to go into emergency with chest pain and you desperately need someone to accurately interpret your ECG) leads to the same level of impairment as being legally drunk.
- Changes in perception. Problems that may be entirely soluble when you are well rested often feel insurmountable when you are sleep-deprived.
- Cognitive impairment, memory disturbance, and difficulty learning new tasks. An Israeli study found that fourth grade and sixth grade kids who were deprived of just one hour of sleep a night for a few weeks experienced a significant drop-off in cognitive test scores of

attention and memory and in school performance. What's perhaps even more striking is that a fourth grade kid who was made to go to bed an hour early and thus got an extra hour of sleep a night soon experienced a sharp and quick spike in performance to that of a fifth or even sixth grade level. (Hey, these are Jewish kids, so they're all undoubtedly geniuses—according to their grandparents, anyway.) In another study, students who regularly went to bed late were found to have grade point averages (a measure of performance in university that has been grossly inflated over the past three decades) significantly lower than those students who got to sleep on time. And in another study, Harvard researchers showed that a new skill was more easily retained in people's memory banks if they slept well that night.

- Mood impairment, which can manifest itself as despair, hopelessness, and depression.
- Improper working of the "oops" center (see chapter 6). Not only do people make more mistakes when they are tired, they are also not as quick to identify them as obvious errors.
- Behavior problems in kids. According to a few studies, some wired kids and kids who seem to have mild forms of attention-deficit disorder and hyperactivity may actually be sleep-deprived.
- Irritability.
- Lower pain threshold.
- Social problems: in school, at work, in relationships.
- Visual problems.
- Coordination problems.
- Accidents. Every kind of accident occurs more frequently in sleep-deprived individuals (see below).

Chronic sleep deprivation has been linked to all sorts of health disorders, including:

- Increased overall mortality. Several studies have shown that difficulty falling asleep is linked to an earlier death.
- Heart disease. Short bouts of sleep deprivation have been linked to spikes in blood pressure and altered blood factors associated with inflammation.

- Diabetes and impaired insulin sensitivity. One study found that chronic sleep deprivation (average 6.5 hours per night) was as damaging to insulin sensitivity as other risk factors, such as obesity and lack of exercise.
- Obesity. Studies have shown that sleep loss has a negative effect on hormones (no surprise, if hormones are geared to a 24-hour day-and-night clock, which they are), carbohydrate metabolism, and perhaps appetite, too, all of which lead to a greater risk of putting on weight. When I read this to my son, he tried to convince me that instead of exercising and dieting, he was just going to sleep more to lose weight. Nice try, don't you think?
- Altered immunity. Chronic insomnia has been linked to lower numbers of circulating infection-fighting cells.

Depending on your point of view, by the way, there is one benefit of being sleep-deprived: apparently, libido jumps. Well, if you can't sleep, anyway...

Treatment
So what can you do if you find that getting to sleep is becoming a drag? It all starts, the experts say, with proper sleep hygiene, which doesn't mean washing your hands and brushing your teeth before going to bed, though that's certainly a good idea. Rather, it refers to doing things to make sleep easier and eliminating activities that have nothing to do with sleep:

- Go to bed at roughly the same time every night. This practice is not only good for your health but also good for your marriage. My wife invariably falls asleep around 9 PM, whereas I have always gone to bed near midnight. And that, ladies and gents, may be the real secret to our 33 years of wedded bliss.
- Get up at the same time every morning.
- Try to wind down and relax before going to bed.
- Don't eat too close to bedtime. Heavy meals, especially, interfere with sleep, as do any foods that increase acid reflux.
- Don't drink anything, either. One study found that a large number of men referred for evaluation of a sleep problem actually had a

prostate problem instead. When this condition was corrected and the subjects no longer had to get up several times a night to pee, their sleep quality improved immensely. And it's not just old men who pee too much at night. Anyone taking diuretics, anyone who eats a lot fruit, women with some bladder conditions, and most light sleepers also do.

- Avoid exercise close to bedtime. Yes, exercise during the day does often dramatically improve sleep quality (studies show that competitive runners usually sleep better after races), but exercise is also a stimulating activity (at least, it should be) and therefore should not take place close to the time you want to go to sleep. Some people may sleep better after exercising, but they are a small minority. For most of us, exercise too close to bedtime helps keep us up, and yes, sex can be a stimulating exercise, too (or so I've been told).

- Reserve the bedroom only for sex and sleep and not for (and I swear the experts all use this example) paying the bills. Trust me folks: anyone who pays the bills in bed needs a lot more help than merely some suggestions about his sleep hygiene.

- Avoid stimulants near bedtime. Coffee, alcohol, and nicotine are all stimulants, so that glass of wine before and that cigarette after are bound to keep you up longer. May be worth it, though. Remember, too, that chocolate and some drugs contain caffeine. A special word about alcohol: for the purposes of sleep, it sucks. Yes, alcohol produces drowsiness, but the sleep that alcohol leads to is the sleep of the damned, not to mention that it makes sleep apnea much worse and interacts negatively with other drugs you may be taking to help you sleep from time to time.

- Avoid naps (maybe). The jury is still out on the benefits of napping (because in some people they can interfere with nighttime sleep), even though some studies show that short afternoon naps improve work and school performance. On the plus side of napping, some very famous and successful people are or were quite notorious nappers, such as Winston Churchill and my wife, Phyllis, who attributes her business success to two things: her frequent naps and her husband (she listens gravely to all my suggestions and then does the complete opposite; I don't mind because it's made her business a huge success).

- Make sure the bedroom is conducive to sleep. It's clearly much easier to fall asleep in a room that's dark and quiet and at the right temperature, though when two people share a bedroom, finding the "right" temperature is not always easy. Phyllis, for example, prefers arctic conditions, whereas I am much more normal and prefer a semitropical climate; we've compromised (I often sleep in a parka).
- Try to relax yourself in bed. British researchers claim that thinking of a tranquil scene is probably a whole lot better for you than counting "the same old dirty sheep," advice that I have taken to heart. Now when I can't sleep, I no longer count the number of anti-American Canadians I know but just think of a tranquil, relaxing scene instead, such as a meadow full of all those Stanley Cups the Maple Leafs haven't won.
- If you don't fall asleep in 20 to 30 minutes, get up and do something else for a few minutes; just lying there and steaming about why you can't get to sleep is usually counterproductive. But be sure to do things that won't make you more aroused. A good rule is to listen to whatever is on NPR or the CBC.
- Although the experts rarely mention this, if you're having trouble sleeping, you might try kicking your kitty or your hound out of the bedroom. A survey for the Mayo Clinic Sleep Disorders Center found that 22 percent of allegedly normal people slept with a pet on the bed, even though over half of those pet owners felt the pet was disturbing their sleep (many pets snore!). So be firm and put the snoring schnauzer in the shed where he belongs so that you don't end up dog-tired the next day.
- You can also try one of many recommended home remedies, the most popular being a warm glass of milk. Milk contains lots of the amino acid L-tryptophan, which is commonly said to be a sleep inducer, and is more easily released when milk is warm or hot (careful, though). By the way, turkey also contains L-tryptophan, which is why Thanksgiving meals—turkeys talking turkey—are so sleep-provoking. (And here you always thought it was family stories that led to instant snoozeville.)
- Over-the-counter drugs that are commonly used include the older generation of antihistamines, diphenhydramine (Benadryl, Nytol

Extra Strength, others) and dimenhydrinate (more commonly known as Gravol), which have the side effect of causing drowsiness. They are certainly effective in some people, but are also known to produce excessive daytime drowsiness (as well as dry mouth, headaches, and gastrointestinal side effects), so be very careful if you have to drive the morning after taking one of them. Curiously, these drugs can also cause what is known as a reciprocal effect; rather than leading to sedation, they can produce agitation and excessive arousal in some people. Also, these drugs can lead to difficulty emptying the bladder, so anyone with an enlarging prostate should be careful about taking them. As with any medications, be aware that these can also react with other drugs.

- Commonly used herbal remedies include valerian, chamomile tea, verbena, and a host of others that are heavily promoted by your neighborhood and clearly well-rested health food store worker. But just because something is "natural," don't be seduced into thinking it's completely risk-free; find out all you can about the potential side effects of these herbs before using them.
- One self-remedy I've never been impressed with, by the way, is melatonin. I know that melatonin is supposed to work, but it's never worked for me. If it works for you, however, who am I to talk you out of your placebo? Oops.

For more chronic sleep problems, there are a host of self-help therapies, including relaxation techniques, meditation, yoga, and so on, all of which are geared to reducing arousal. Other forms of sleep therapy that involve the services of health professionals include:

- Sleep restriction, in which the sadistic therapist restricts you to staying in bed only for the exact amount of time you usually spend asleep (say five to six hours), and once you get to the point that you are asleep the entire time you're in bed, the therapist then allows you gradually more time in bed, which presumably will also be sleep time.
- Cognitive behavior therapy, in which the insomniac learns what's been keeping her awake. ("You mean it's those damn bills? Why

didn't I think of that? Gee, you're worth every cent of that $3,000 I paid you, Doc.") Then she presumably relearns to fall asleep on time.

- Hypnotic sedatives. Hypnotic sedatives include the benzodiazepines (drugs that have been around for years) such as lorazepam (Ativan) and triazolam (Halcion), as well as some of the newer non-benzodiazepines such as zopiclone (Imovane) and zaleplon (Starnoc in Canada, Sonata in the U.S.). All of them are effective at producing sleep, though they differ significantly in how long they take to put you to sleep and how long they remain active and keep circulating in your bloodstream (the longer these drugs remain active, the longer you feel drowsy), so it's important to make sure that you get the right drug for your needs.

The most common side effects of these drugs are:

- Next-day drowsiness and fatigue
- Nausea
- Dizziness
- Headache
- In some people, a reciprocal effect (arousal instead of sedation)
- A bad taste (zopiclone)

They can also:

- Cause disturbances in memory (but then what doesn't?)
- Disrupt attention
- Make sleep apnea worse, which is why it's important to come up with an accurate diagnosis for the specific sleep problem you have
- Interact with other medications and substances such as alcohol

If you are prescribed any of these meds, or if you are taking a self-prescribed over-the-counter remedy from your local health store, always keep in mind my wife's very useful bedroom mantra: start low, go slow. So always start with the lowest dose you figure might work (one-quarter of a standard hypnotic dose is enough to induce two nights' sleep in my wife) and increase the dose only if necessary.

Also, always bear in mind that these drugs produce both tolerance and dependence. Tolerance means that if you stay on a drug, your body gets used to it, so you will need more and more of it to get the same effect. Dependence means that these drugs are habit-forming, so if you're on them for a while, you will suffer withdrawal symptoms if you decide to stop taking them (as well as rebound insomnia, or a sudden worsening of the exact problem you started taking the drug for in the first place). So it's not a good idea to take any of these meds for long.

How long is too long? There are no formulas, but if you're getting up to two weeks, you should definitely put a lid on it. This also applies to over-the-counter remedies.

If you've taken meds for a while, it's usually best to gradually taper off—take half a pill for a bit, then a quarter of a pill, and so on, till you're completely off.

◆ ———————————————————————————————— ◆

A SPECIAL CAUTION

I want to single out one particular problem related to lack of sleep because it's such an important killer: the risk of being involved in a motor vehicle accident when you're drowsy. An American study found that someone who sleeps six to seven hours a night is twice as likely to be involved in a motor vehicle accident as is someone who sleeps eight hours a night. New Zealand researchers report that sleepy drivers are eight times as likely as rested drivers to be involved in a motor vehicle accident, and that a dead man driving—someone who sleeps only five hours a night—is five times as likely to be involved in such an accident. Overall, American authorities estimate that sleep deprivation accounts for over one million motor vehicle accidents a year, which is more accidents than are caused by either alcohol use or substance abuse. Lack of sleep is especially lethal when combined with recreational drug use or use of alcohol.

The really scary thing is that most sleep-deprived individuals involved in accidents don't even recognize (or acknowledge) how tired they were before the crash or how great a danger they posed. In one survey, 20 percent of American adult drivers admitted to falling asleep while driving (mea culpa, mea culpa, although never since I left university and those late-night BS sessions where we were planning how we were going to change the world; nearly all of us became middle-class health professionals, by the way), and 50 percent admitted to driving while "drowsy" at least once.

The good news, though, is that lots of companies are working on devices to help wake up drowsy drivers, at least until they can make it to a rest stop to get some shut-eye. Apparently, one device can detect when eyelids are droopy, and another gadget shoots questions at a driver and grades him on the answers. (When you combine those devices, by the way, you end up with what they call a wife. A wife is an amazingly useful multipurpose gadget to have—even better than a Swiss Army Knife.) If these devices detect any problem, they apparently kick in with some kind of wake-up tool: the radio blares away, the windows roll down, or the air-conditioning starts blasting—some gadgets even shoot cold water in the driver's face and yell at him. (See? I told you how multipurpose they are.)

◆ ———————————————————————————— ◆

SNORING

Snoring is sound produced during sleep when breathing is partially obstructed. There are few accurate statistics on snoring because, after all, it generally takes an observer to determine if someone else is snoring, and what might be a snore to one person is a peaceful, restful sigh to another. That said, it's commonly accepted that 40 percent of men snore, as do 30 percent of women (though when it comes to admitting that they snore, the score is quite different: 40 percent of men and zero percent of women admit to snoring), with the elderly more likely to snore than the young.

Snoring occurs when the soft tissues in the throat vibrate over airways that have narrowed, usually when tissues at the back or sides of the throat "collapse" as they relax, or when some structure—adenoids, tonsils, uvula, or the tongue falling back—narrows the passage. At least one study claims that this is most likely to occur in "round-headed" people as opposed to people with long, thin faces.

Clearly, anything that increases the narrowing of the air passages or lowers the muscle tone of the tissues in the back of the throat can make snoring worse.

Among the most common factors are the following:

- Alcohol
- Medications such as sleeping pills and antihistamines
- Colds
- Hay fever
- Swollen tonsils and adenoids
- Obesity
- Smoking

Snoring has long been viewed as no more than a nuisance, especially to the person forced to listen to the rumble. More recently, though, snoring has been seen to be part of a continuum that ends with sleep apnea (see below). That is, snoring is caused by partial obstruction of the air passages and sleep apnea is caused by complete obstruction of the airways. Thus, snoring, too, has been independently linked to negative health consequences:

- Relationship problems. In one survey, 50 percent of British couples claimed that snoring was a major cause of arguments, 25 percent said that snoring was playing havoc with their sex lives (well, wouldn't you be upset if your partner snored during sex?), and 40 percent said that snoring had a negative impact on their lives.
- Higher risk of strokes. An Italian study found that even if loud snorers were not diagnosed with sleep apnea, they still had a higher risk of stroke than nonsnorers.
- Diabetes. In the Nurses' Health Study, snoring nurses (the mind does boggle) were twice as likely to end up with Type 2 diabetes.
- High blood pressure.
- Chronic daily headaches, especially when snoring is part of obstructive sleep apnea.

What can you do about snoring? Well, if you're the captive listener, you can:

- Learn to love it.
- Get earplugs.

- Kick the snorer. Snoring is usually much worse when the snorer sleeps on her—excuse me, I mean, of course, his—back (the relaxed tissues flop around more easily). Also, when a snorer changes position, the snoring is usually interrupted, at least for a while.
- When all else fails, move out.

For the snorer, therapy includes:

- First checking to see if you have sleep apnea or any correctable condition such as allergies or polyps.
- Getting down to a more normal weight.
- Avoiding factors that make snoring worse, such as alcohol.
- Using anti-snoring devices that try to enlarge the opening of the upper air passages in the throat.
- Having surgery. There are several surgical techniques to ease snoring, but as always with surgery, it's buyer beware. Not only is surgery permanent (you want to be really, really sure that you won't be worse off afterward), but also snoring is often due to several tissue abnormalities, not just the one being worked on by the surgeons.

SLEEP APNEA

Although there are over 80 recognized sleep disorders (bedwetting, restless leg syndrome, fear of dreaming about Don Cherry, etc.), sleep apnea is perhaps the one most linked with lifestyle. In sleep apnea, sleep is interrupted by periodic cessation of breathing, which scares the hell out of the bed partner but does nothing to the apneic individual, who goes snoringly on his way (most people with sleep apnea are men) when his breathing starts up again. These stop-breathing spells can last from 10 seconds to—yikes!—over a minute.

There are two kinds of sleep apnea:

- Central sleep apnea (CSA) is caused by a problem either in the brain or in the heart. CSA constitutes about 10 percent of sleep apnea cases.
- Obstructive sleep apnea (OSA) occurs because something temporarily blocks the breathing passages. OSA accounts for roughly 90 percent of cases.

Risk factors for sleep apnea include:

- Obesity.
- Being male, though a third of sleep apnea patients are women.
- Having a thick neck. One study found that OSA is much more prevalent in NFL linebackers, for example, than in the general population.
- Having a long, thin pharynx.
- Old age. As always, this condition is more common in the elderly, but several studies have found that sleep apnea is surprisingly common in kids, too, especially in those who snore.
- Menopause.

Obstructive sleep apnea can be worsened by anything that relaxes neck tone, including:

- Alcohol use.
- The use of sleeping medications.
- Sleeping on the back.
- Smoking.

How do you know you have sleep apnea? You usually don't, because loud snoring alone is not enough to diagnose this condition adequately. Sleep researchers in northern Wales are working on a portable device that monitors noise levels and can apparently identify the difference between "normal" snoring and snoring due to sleep apnea.

Until that device is commercially available, though, the next best aid in figuring out whether you might have OSA is if your sleeping mate has ever said, "Hey, I thought you nearly bought the farm last night," and she was clearly not referring to the fact that you had made a good purchase on a few cows and some pasture. Rather, she was referring to the fact that you had stopped breathing while asleep and she had seen you gasp a few times before resuming your normal snoring. Intermittent bouts of cessation of breathing, gasping, returning to normal breathing, another episode of cessation of breathing, more gasping, and so on can occur frequently throughout the night (up to 60 times an hour, in the worst cases), and the remarkable thing is that the snorer is blissfully unaware that it is happening.

So if you sleep alone—or, I suppose, if you sleep next to someone who also has sleep apnea so that she, too, has no idea that it's abnormal to stop breathing and gasp over and over during sleep—the most common signs and symptoms include:

- Unrefreshing sleep, so that you never feel as if you get a good night's sleep.
- Excessive daytime sleepiness.
- A strong history of snoring.
- Being overweight.
- Chronic morning headaches. One study found that 84 percent of patients with chronic morning headaches who also snore have sleep apnea.

Why does it matter to know if you have sleep apnea? Because it can kill you, and while killing you, it might take out a lot of other people at the same time. Sleep apnea is related to a much higher risk of being involved in accidents. In several European countries, including Spain, the U.K., and France, sleep apnea patients must get treatment or else lose their driver's license (clearly, in France, people with sleep apnea are considered more dangerous than chronic alcoholics, which is why you have to love that country—*zut alors!*).

Sleep apnea has also been linked with:

- Higher blood pressure. High blood pressure is present in more than half the patients who suffer from sleep apnea, and some experts think that up to 40 percent of people who have high blood pressure also have undiagnosed sleep apnea.
- Higher risk of strokes.
- Higher risk of heart disease. A small study that tracked middle-aged men for nine years found that those with sleep apnea were more likely to be diagnosed with some kind of heart problem and, in fact, that sleep apnea was a better predictor of eventual heart disease problems than any other risk factor.
- Higher risk of heart failure, cardiac rhythm disturbances, and blood clots.

- Higher risk of diabetes, in part, I suppose, because both these conditions are related to being overweight.
- Brain abnormalities. An interesting study found that 40 percent of patients with sleep apnea had stuttered during childhood, raising the possibility that both were caused by some type of early brain injury.
- Dementia. Individuals who carry a gene that raises their risk of Alzheimer's disease are also more likely to suffer from sleep apnea.
- Significantly more complications following surgery.
- A negative impact on psychological well-being: higher rates of depression, marital discord, social problems, or chronic anxiety.
- Higher rates of GERD. An excellent study from Duke University shows that treating sleep apnea also relieves nighttime GERD symptoms.
- Lower levels of testosterone at night, and you know where that takes you, eh? Shopping.

Because sleep quality is so poor, sleep apnea is also related to:

- Poorer concentration.
- Poorer performance of tasks.
- In kids, behavior problems and a higher risk of being diagnosed with ADHD (attention-deficit hyperactivity disorder). If you have a youngster who snores and who acts out, it might be worth getting his sleep assessed. You might also have his tonsils and adenoids evaluated, and if those are to blame for poor sleep, then get them yanked out. Hey, that's certainly better than a lifetime supply of Ritalin.

Treatment of sleep apnea is essential. Not only does successful treatment lead to a significant improvement in quality of life, but studies also show that successful treatment results in lower risks of complications, such as heart failure and stroke. Treatment obviously starts with lifestyle changes, such as losing weight and keeping alcohol intake to a minimum. A study published in the *Journal of the American Medical Association* looked at 700 people with sleep apnea for over four years and found that weight loss of 10 percent of body weight (6.8 kilograms [15 pounds] in a 68-kilogram [150-pound] person is a difficult goal but not unattainable—especially when your life's at stake) led to significant improvement in symptoms, and presumably to a significant lowering of future health risks, too.

If the lifestyle adjustments don't work, the next step should be a device known as a Continuous Positive Airway Pressure, or CPAP, machine (a pump attached to a mask or nose plugs that keep the airways open by blowing air through a tube into the breathing passageway). The problem with CPAP is that lots of sleep apnea patients don't like it, and 20 to 50 percent will not tolerate it. An alternative is choosing one of a host of dental devices on the market that are supposed to keep breathing passages from blocking as easily, and there are studies to show that they work for mild sleep apnea, although I haven't seen studies yet showing that they lower the ultimate risk of stroke.

If none of those therapies work, then several kinds of surgery can be useful, such as cutting away part of the upper palate, though even these procedures are not nearly as successful as was once hoped. Finally, an interesting study published recently concluded that in a small group of patients with sleep apnea, the antidepressant Remeron led to a significant improvement, including fewer periods of stopped breathing.

9

Stress

You Say Pussycat, I Say Tiger

Prevention always supersedes treatment in importance.
DR. ANDREW WEIL, *Eight Weeks to Optimum Health*

The lion and the calf shall lie down together but the calf
won't get much sleep.
WOODY ALLEN, *Without Feathers*

I'VE TOLD YOU several times that I am a method writer. While writing about alcohol, I drank wine; while writing about nutrition, I ate continuously; while writing about smoking, I routinely walked by government buildings to catch the drift of passive smoke emitted by the workers huddled outside; during the chapter on exercise, I took time off regularly to work out. As for the upcoming chapter on sex, well, there's only so much about me you ought to know—or want to know, I'm sure.

I was, however, hoping to deviate from my plan while writing about stress, but I'm afraid I didn't, and in fact this chapter nearly did me in. You see, this was the last chapter I worked on, and it was way, way overdue, and my editor kept calling to ask how I was doing (she's too polite to have asked me directly if I was working on the book), so without meaning to, I reacquainted myself with acute stress much more than had been my intention in taking on this project.

Indeed, one of the earliest and worst things I discovered in researching this chapter was a study that instantly got me reaching for tranquilizers: U.S. governors elected at a young age have a significantly shorter life span than governors first elected when they're older. The implication is clear: the younger you are when you amount to something important, the sooner you're likely to say hello to your maker.

"I'm really nervous now," I lamented to my wife, "because I was only 23 when I graduated from medical school."

"Don't worry, dear," she cooed reassuringly. "You're OK—you haven't really achieved anything significant in your life."

What a woman, eh? She has that special knack for making me feel much better no matter how down I get.

What Is Stress?

Hans Selye, the godfather of stress research, defined stress as the "nonspecific response of any organism to any pressure or demand on it," meaning two very important things: (1) even an amoeba (or a lawyer) can feel stress, and (2) stress is usually nothing more than what we make out of something that's confronting us—"stress" is our own "response" to something we perceive as a threat or a challenge.

Take, for example, someone who suddenly sees my malamute, Big Louie, running full-tilt off the leash toward him in the park. That person may (1) turn tail and try to outrun Big Louie ("flight response"), (2) stop dead in his tracks to yell at me to put my huge dog back on his leash ("fight response"), (3) welcome Louie's attention and pet him and say, "Nice doggy, nice doggy, want a cookie? Down doggy, don't bite my finger" ("right response"), or (4) ignore Louie and continue smelling the flowers (another "right response").

Two people confronted by the same situation often perceive that situation entirely differently and consequently react differently. One person may experience an intense stress response because she has evaluated that situation as one that poses a threat or danger to her, whereas the other person might just go along as if nothing important is happening. An event, an animal, a person, a question, or even an audit is not usually a "stressor" in and of itself (actually, I take that back about the audit). Rather, it's the observer's evaluation and assessment that defines a stressor and assesses its threat. As wise men say, "One man's pussycat is another man's tiger."

What, then, determines how you react? Most important is your history—what you have learned; how you have reacted in the past to similar circumstances; how you were brought up to deal with such events; where you are now in your life even, perhaps, according to a recent study; how your mother handled you and treated you when you were an infant. Also, your state of mind, your mood, your fatigue level, and anything to do with how you feel at that moment are very important in helping determine whether something acts as a stressor for you or not.

And so is personality. Take, for example, a familiar source of significant stress for many people: driving in traffic. A recent British survey found that traffic jams are the biggest self-assessed cause of daily stress in most people's lives.

So say you're going to a meeting, and the traffic is really bad. Now, you clearly have only two choices in how to react. You can say to yourself, "Hey, this is really no big deal. Tomorrow is another day. There's always Tara. I'm not in that much of a rush, anyway, and if this deal I'm already late for doesn't come through, then hey, another one will surely come along in its place, and besides, I don't really need that job, anyway, so I might as well relax because this, too, shall pass. Amen."

Or you can veer off to a side street to avoid the interminable lights that you know will inevitably turn red just as you approach them, not to mention the hundreds of imbecile pedestrians who have the chutzpah to cross the road just as you get to their crosswalk, and, of course, as you turn onto that quiet side street, another car—nearly always an Echo or a Tercel—blocks your way as the driver, some old person wearing a hat, or worse, a woman, slowly navigates that street looking for an address that is surely only imaginary. This threat to your well-being provokes you to blow your horn and yell at that slow driver (though she won't hear you, of course, because she's too busy checking the addresses and applying makeup) and seethe.

If you're the kind of person who responds in the first manner—with placidity and an even temper or resignation to the inevitability that "shit happens, man, deal with it"—this kind of event does not act as a stressor for you, and it's likely that you will be blessed with tranquility, peace, and low blood pressure throughout your life (though you will also be late for many meetings, but then, hey, you're not the kind of person who cares about that). It also means you're a saintly Type B (see below).

If you respond normally, however—that is, in the second manner— then you are the kind of person who is bombarded with showers of minor daily unavoidable irritations that become instant stressors for you. It also means that you are a Type A personality, a term coined a few decades ago by cardiologists Dr. Meyer Friedman and Dr. Ray Rosenman for the typical hurry-up, intensely competitive, overachieving, impatient, perfectionist, often hostile first-born son of immigrant parents. Actually, I lie. Being a first-born immigrant son was not part of that first description of Type A personality (though it certainly fits every one of us).

In contrast to Type A's, Friedman and Rosenman claimed that the other response—"I should get out and help her find the right address, but maybe I'll just take a snooze first"—was more likely to emanate from a Type B personality, the kind of person who doesn't care at all if the meeting is held today or tomorrow or ever.

Friedman and Rosenman suggested that Type A's were significantly more at risk of premature heart attacks than Type B's, findings that were confirmed by other researchers. It subsequently became widely accepted that harried and hurry-up Type A's were much more prone to the deleterious effects of stress, especially cardiac disease, than those let-it-be Type B's.

That simple view has become considerably more complicated, however, as studies have revealed that not all Type A's are at equally raised risk of deleterious health consequences as a result of their personalities. Some Type A's do very well, thank you very much, because we are so determined to do everything correctly (well, we can't expect our Type B brothers to do it for us, eh?) that many of us end up leading very healthy lifestyles from which we benefit greatly. We exercise a lot (to the exact minute, of course, noting and charting every minute change in blood pressure and heart rate), we eat properly (chomping on exact servings of each specific food group every day), we drink exactly 227 milliliters (8 fluid ounces) of red wine every evening, and so on, which translates, as you might expect, into much better health outcomes for many of us. Moreover, some of us love challenging situations because we can measure ourselves against them, so we don't respond to many of these potential threats by mounting a stress response.

In contrast, some Type B's simply can't be bothered to worry about doing healthy lifestyle things, because, "Hey, man, what's the big deal, eh?" And sometimes not responding to a potential threat may not be the wisest response. It surely stands to reason, for example, that many a saber-toothed tiger ended up munching on the carcass of many a Type B who hadn't felt the need to run quite as fast as his Type A brother.

So over the past few years that simple view of Type A and Type B has been refined considerably, and most experts now believe that the danger to health comes more from specific "negative" personality traits and other elements of one's emotional well-being than from overall personality. For example, "extreme impatience" is now thought by many to be a particularly damaging personality characteristic (not all Type A's are extremely impatient; some of us have learned to just grit our teeth and wait), a trait that medical people refer to as time urgency/impatience, or TUI. For people with TUI, no one, especially your wife, is ever on time or can ever get anything done fast enough to satisfy your majesty.

"We should have left 20 minutes ago."

"But it doesn't start for an hour, and anyway, it's only across the street."

"So?"

How bad is TUI for you? Well, one great study found that over a period of 13 years, a TUI trait was linked to twice the risk of eventual high blood pressure. Curiously, this link held true for men only, a discrepancy the authors were unable to explain. (I can explain it easily, though: women never mind being late. You're welcome.)

But perhaps the most malignant personality trait is hostility. "What is hostility?" you ask. Well, hostility is like modern art—it's not easy to describe, but you sure know it when you run into it. It can include cynicism, a lack of trust, sarcasm, and, perhaps especially, a temper that goes off at the drop of a hat. A fascinating study of 1,000 men found that over

40 years, those men judged to be most hostile in their youth were three times as likely to be diagnosed with heart disease and up to five times as likely to suffer a heart attack before age 55 than were their more placid brothers. In another intriguing study from the Henry Ford Hospital in Detroit, men who were labeled as "cranky" were significantly more likely to be diagnosed with heart disease.

Another American study found that men who scored high on the scale for hostility were eventually much more likely to suffer a heart attack and concluded that a personality test was an exceptionally accurate screening tool for eventual heart disease. The only risk factor that was a better predictor of future heart disease was a low level of HDL.

As for women, in the HERS (Heart and Estrogen/Progestin Replacement) study of postmenopausal women, hostile women had double the risk of dying from a heart attack compared with their more accepting sisters. In fact, their "bad attitude" was deemed to be a worse risk to these women's hearts than smoking, high blood pressure, and abnormal lipid levels.

And hostility is just as harmful to the young as it is to adults. A recent study found that "hostile" adolescents were more likely to develop the metabolic syndrome (see chapter 5) over a three-year follow-up study than were their less hostile peers.

What Leads to Stress?
So far, I've made light of stressors by using examples that may be considered minor by many of you, such as traffic jams. But stress can be induced by anything you can't control, varying from minor irritants to larger, more ominous events, such as war, the loss of a job, disease-carrying mosquitoes, or kids not behaving the way we did, that is, perfect in every way. Anything that causes us to feel that our control is ebbing or has been taken away can lead us to suffer the health effects of stress-related illness.

After Scud missiles started raining down in Israel during the first Gulf War, for example, the heart attack rate went up significantly for the following week. After September 11, 2001, the heart attack rate also spiked dramatically in New York, as did the rate of heart rhythm abnormalities (doctors detected a significant rise in arrhythmias in people wearing implanted defibrillators). These risks stayed elevated for several weeks after September 11, because for once, New Yorkers, those quintessential control freaks, felt a lack of adequate control over their environment.

We can't do much to control the fact that we live in a world where Saudi Arabian terrorists—excuse me, oppressed, middle-class, educated, virgin-seeking liberation-fighters from no singled-out grievance group or specific country—hijack planes and ram them into buildings and kill innocent civilians. Nor can you do much about your teenage daughter when she suddenly springs on you her new tattoo and latest-boyfriend, Spike, the 54-year-old head of the local Hells Angels gang. Some types of stressors are just beyond our ability to control.

Far too often, however, most of us activate our stress response to minor events that are not inherently dangerous or threatening, events that may result in a continual and prolonged activation of our stress response, and that's where the real trouble lies.

What Happens When You Are Under Stress?
The stress response, also known as the "fight or flight" reaction, is a very complex cascade of inner changes. Adrenaline and other stress hormones are released into the bloodstream; the senses are heightened ("Did I just hear you say what I think you said?"); blood pressure, heart rate, and respiratory rate spike ("I'm so worked up, my heart's beating faster than a one-armed carpet-cleaner"); the liver releases energy fuel in the form of glucose and fats; blood is diverted from peripheral organs (the skin, intestines, etc.) to the organs of action (brain, muscles); the blood becomes "thicker" in order to clot more easily should you suffer a bleed; the immune system is activated; and many other changes take place.

Clearly, however, this state of high alert is not healthy if it continues unabated for too long or if it becomes too intense, so one of the "stress hormones" also has the job of dampening both the stress reaction and the activation of the immune system. ("OK, the Cossacks are gone. Let's eat.")

In the short term, this interrelated activation of the nervous system, the immune system, and the endocrine system is no problem and may even be a help, because there are still modern-day equivalents of saber-toothed tigers out there ("Feet, don't fail me now."). Also, it often feels good to become more aroused, as, say, by a good poker hand or a designer dress suddenly marked down. But often that fight-or-flight reaction produces more harm than benefit, since most modern-day stressors are of a minor nature that don't require such an intense or prolonged response. Further, the more often this response is triggered and the longer each individual reaction lasts (that is, the more chronic stress we're under), the more our bodies wear down as a consequence.

As well, we live in a society that produces unreasonable demands on many of us—too many jobs with too little control, such as those of a woman in her forties who works outside the home, takes care of an aging parent, shepherds three kids through adolescence, and nurtures a husband who's often the most immature of the lot (as with Woody Allen, there is nothing autobiographical in any of this, I assure you—and, anyway, we only have two kids). This imbalance in our lives also exacts a significant stress-related toll on us.

What Does Repeated Stress Do to You?

Some of the psychological changes associated with stress include:

- Irritability
- Anxiety
- Depression
- Mood swings
- Phobias

Some of the physical symptoms associated with stress include:

- Pain
- Fatigue
- Sleep disruption
- Aggravation of pre-existing conditions

But beyond producing symptoms, chronic stress also leads to deleterious health consequences. One of the most harmful effects related to chronic (and acute) stress is dying prematurely from cardiovascular disease. In the beautifully named study known as MRFIT (Multiple Risk

Factor Intervention Trial), those men most likely to die over 16 years of follow-up were men who were either divorced (bad news for those who think divorce is *supposed* to decrease stress levels) or under the most stress. In another study, the researchers concluded that mental stress can trigger fatal heart problems in people with pre-existing heart disease (many of whom don't even know they have a wonky heart, of course). In an eight-year study of over 30,000 Japanese women, those women who reported the most stress were the most likely to die of a stroke or heart attack by the end of the study. And another 13-year study found that people claiming to be under high levels of chronic stress were significantly more likely to suffer a fatal stroke by the end of the study.

How does chronic stress affect the cardiovascular system?

- Many studies have shown that chronic stress is related to higher blood pressure. In one study, just thinking about a stressful event led to a jump in blood pressure in a group of students, and the longer the students ruminated on the event, the longer their blood pressures stayed elevated.
- Stress may lead to less flexible arteries.
- Chronic stress seems to lead to greater storage of fat as abdominal fat.
- Stress may impede the body's ability to clear fats from the bloodstream.
- Chronic stress might even lead to unhealthy lipid levels.
- Stress raises the levels of chemicals associated with inflammation.
- Perhaps most important, chronically stressed people tend to have the unhealthiest lifestyles.

This link between stress and cardiovascular health (or lack of it), however, is not always as clear-cut as might seem.

A study of U.S. army personnel found that stressed-out (depressed, anxious, hostile) hypochondriacs — that is, people like my father and my brother and my two sons (but not, oddly enough, like me), who think they're sick but really aren't — not only were no more likely to end up with cardiovascular disease than nonstressed-out people but were actually the "least likely" to end up with hardened arteries. In a 20-year study of Scottish men published in the *British Medical Journal*, men who developed heart disease invariably thought that stress had played a large role in their getting sick, but when the data were looked at objectively, the researchers concluded that stress actually played no role in the development of heart disease in these men. That is probably because the most stressed men were also the most well-off and the ones most likely to be doing the right things to mitigate their risk of having a heart attack.

Besides its effects on the cardiovascular system, chronic stress also has other negative health consequences:

- It adversely affects our hormonal and endocrine systems. One study found that stress in marriage was related to double the risk of diabetes, making it more of a risk factor than a poor family history. Conversely, in those who already have diabetes, learning to manage stress can improve blood glucose levels.
- Nearly every disease or disability can be related to higher chronic stress levels, so that even if stress doesn't cause a specific medical problem, chronic stress can certainly worsen the symptoms of that problem.
- Stress can alter our immune systems. Studies show that people who judge themselves to be under lots of stress tend to get more colds, and the colds tend to last longer than in people not equally stressed. Other studies have shown that raised stress levels can reduce the level of antibodies your body can manufacture, which can have a negative effect on the protection that vaccinations such as pneumonia vaccine, flu vaccine, and hepatitis B vaccine offer. So if you have to get a shot, such as a flu shot, try to get it when your stress levels are as low as you can possibly get them. On that ubiquitous other hand, though, "good" stress—stress that isn't seen to pose a danger or risk—might actually boost the immune system.
- Chronic stress has been shown to shrink the hippocampus, the area of the brain crucial to the development of memory.
- Asthma is said to be worsened by stress, and a Canadian study linked stress with higher risks of COPD.
- Digestive system disorders such as GERD, diarrhea, constipation, and irritable bowel syndrome are all worsened by stress.

- Depression and other mood disorders, Alzheimer's disease and other forms of dementia are all exacerbated by stress.
- Studies have concluded that stress can lead to poorer skin functioning, leading to more problems with eczema, psoriasis, and a host of other skin conditions.

STRESS AND CANCER

One major health problem that cannot be clearly attributable to the effects of chronic stress is any type of cancer, even though most people who get the disease blame their stress level at least in part for their illness. Objectively, however, in the usual studies that are supposed to carry muster with physicians, it's been hard to pin down stress as a specific cause of cancer on a par, say, with smoking as a cause of lung cancer.

Chronic stress, however, does make it harder to have a healthy lifestyle, so there must be at least that connection between stress and cancer. Moreover chronic stress certainly worsens a cancer patient's ability to deal with the cancer and its consequences (fatigue, for example, or pain). And finally, controlling stress after cancer is diagnosed will also allow a cancer patient to deal with therapy more easily.

How to Cope

If you're overwhelmed with chronic stress, there are really only a few things to do. First, you must acknowledge that you are indeed not doing a good job of handling what's happening to you. Second, examine your life and figure out what's causing the most stress. Third, after a thorough and honest assessment, figure out what you can do about it. You can't, for example, change your boss, but you might be able to change jobs, even if it means a temporary disruption and some longer-term risk. And remember that a stressful situation will not improve just because you want it to, so you have only three choices: (a) learn to live with it as best you can, (b) try to get it changed, and (c) leave.

Remember, too, that there are no stress-free people in this world, and if you get out of one stressful situation, you may head into another that's even worse. You have to be very honest and really forthright with yourself when you assess what's causing your stress and how much of a toll you're paying for it. Also, take time to evaluate your values and needs. Do you truly need a $60,000 Lexus SUV if it will put you into significant debt? I love my Lexus, by the way. And I'm beginning to tolerate my banker, too.

Fourth, if you feel you must do something to deal with your stress, take the time to figure out what active therapy you want to pursue, and by active therapy, I don't necessarily mean seeing a shrink or a counselor or joining a group of like-minded people. I would also include things like exercise, becoming religious (or the opposite, losing your religion), or taking up a new hobby.

Anything that might help improve your situation or your perception of your situation is an acceptable thing to try. So, for me, there are as many stress-relieving suggestions, mechanisms, and therapies as there are unemployed doubles of Saddam Hussein. Each of them works for some people (that's why people promote them, after all), but none of them work for everyone, or even most people.

But what does the author do, some of you may wonder, before plunging on. I'm sure most of you know what the answer is: I exercise. I use exercise both as an acute stress reliever—I work out whenever I'm feeling really put upon by my family or my jobs, which is why I work out very often—and I use exercise as a chronic stress reliever, by which I mean that I get so much energy and good feelings from working out that I'm certain it's helped me deal with chronic stress over the past few years.

I also do a lot of mental exercise (some would say that I could profit from doing more), such as reading and especially doing puzzles and crosswords, though I've never consciously considered the Sunday *New York Times* crossword to be a stress reliever because I get so frustrated at the America-centricity of the thing. But hey, filling in the blanks for "a pedagogue in a play by Oscar Wilde: two words" (*Miss Prism*) or "a medieval serf" (*esne*) at night in bed brings me a joy like no other (well, almost no other), and I consequently sleep much easier.

But that's me. I don't for a second presume to tell you what to do (yes, I'm a doctor, but remember that this is a new era and we're "partners" now, so the choice you make is entirely up to you). But here's my advice, partner. Exercise is always a great place to start because it's:

- Cheap
- Easy
- Fast
- Non-embarrassing (you don't have to unburden yourself to a running partner; in fact, if you want to keep that partner, you'd better not unburden yourself)
- Social
- Private (no one has to know that you're running because you're fighting with your spouse)

And best of all, exercise has so many other health benefits. That said, lots of people can't or won't exercise, and that's OK, too. (I nearly hit my fingers while typing this to stop myself from saying it.) There are all sorts of other equally beneficial stress-relieving changes you can make in your life.

- Start leading a healthier lifestyle: eat right, avoid toxins, sleep regular hours, and so on, all of which will help you manage better, even if you don't exercise. As I said earlier, it's all to do with control: if you add more control to your life, life itself becomes more manageable.
- Take vacations. In the Framingham Study, women who took regular vacations lowered their risk of suffering a heart attack, while in the MRFIT study, regular vacation-taking was linked to a 20 percent lower risk of death from cardiovascular disease, probably because vacations lower stress levels and also produce a carryover effect that postpones the day that we again allow all the nagging, niggling worries of everyday life to start eating away at us. (Vacations are not always stress-relieving, however. I once took a flight to Paris, during which my young son broke my glasses and spilled red wine on my white shirt, on top of which Air Canada, as usual, lost my luggage, and let me tell you, trying to convince the very skeptical concierge

of an overbooked Parisian *pension* that yes, that wine-reeking man with no luggage and the stain on his shirt and the glasses held together with duct tape really was the Canadian *medecin* who'd originally booked the room led to the downing of several—large—tranquilizers.)

- Pick a social activity or activities to participate in such as a book club or square-dancing lessons. Having friends and a social life, even playing bingo, for crying out loud, has been linked to better health outcomes, in large part because having a rich social life helps keep the brain active ("Is that B-22 or B-12, Mabel?") and helps minimize the effects of stress, even in animals. In one study, male baboons who spent the most time grooming and being groomed by female friends who were not intended sexual partners (it can only be something unique to baboons, I think) had the lowest levels of stress hormones (they also made the best baboon househusbands).

  In humans, it's the same. In the Health Professionals Follow-Up Study, men who were "socially isolated" had a 20 percent greater risk of dying prematurely (they were 80 percent more likely to die of heart disease, and twice as likely to die violent deaths) than men with a lot of friends and a rich social life.

  And a rich social life may be most important as we age. In a study that looked at quite advanced seniors, the ones most likely to still be alive after about five years were those with the most social contacts.

- Pick a meaningful activity to participate in. Volunteering is social and gives you a great sense of being productive and in control. Lots of people, for example, become members of useful organizations such as local playhouses that put on plays that no one attends or canvass for Greenpeace, or take up the mission of Accountants Without Borders, and so on. Most of them don't, of course, attribute their participation to a need to relieve stress, but it's at least part of the reason we do most such things, whether we're conscious of our motivation or not, beyond that we may actually believe in patronless theater or saving the environment; in fact, giving is so good for you that one study concluded that you will gain a health benefit even if you give of yourself only *once* a year;

- Get a pet. Pet owners tend to have lower markers of stress, such as high blood pressures and heart rates, than do people who don't own pets. Pet owners also have better rates of survival after heart attacks (hey, a dog owner can't afford to die—who's going to take care of Skookums?). One intriguing study even concluded that people get much more stress relief from their pets than they do from their spouses. (Dogs are so much less judgmental, right?)
- Get married. When it comes to health matters, married people do much, much better than their unmarried or divorced or widowed peers. In the Health Professionals Follow-Up Study, married men had a significantly lower risk of dying prematurely from any cause than unmarried men. Another study concluded that divorced or separated men were more than twice as likely to commit suicide as were married men, which may come as a shock to most of the married guys reading this, but it's true. One British study concluded that the benefits of marriage are so great for men that being single was a greater risk for dying prematurely than was being a smoker (marriage was also protective for women, but not as much as for men, though on average, they still outlive us by several years, the stress-inducing dears).

COUPLES COPE WITH STRESS BETTER

Why do married folk handle stress better? Lots of reasons:

- Marriage provides love (well, sometimes, anyway). This may make me sound too much like a Sunday morning radio preacher looking for offerings from demented listeners, but love truly has a life-enhancing power. In one study of men with heart disease, those who claimed their wives loved them had half the rate of angina of their unloved brothers.
- Married people take better care of each other. Do you think any man would ever visit a doctor if his wife didn't nag him to go? Husbands take care of their wives, too. One recent study found that men are less resentful than women when their spouse gets sick and requires care.

- Married people generally have lower blood pressures in the presence of their spouse than when they're alone. One study even found lower stress hormone levels in people who claimed to be happily married than in people who were not.
- Marriage is social (well, it's supposed to be, at any rate).
- Never, never underestimate the health value of regular sex.
- Two incomes beat one, though one study found that when a wife's income is higher than her husband's, some men experience that as a stressor. (Not me, though. I love the fact that my wife outearns me and I have been trying to get her to work even more so that I can take more time off.)
- But the number one reason that marriage benefits women (at any rate) is that male underarm sweat can reduce stress in women. One study has shown that women exposed to male underarm sweat claimed to feel less tense and anxious as a result of that exposure. (Well, I've never really understood women.)

◆ ———————————————————————————— ◆

To be fair, the marriage-is-good-for-what-ails-you thing is not nearly as straightforward as I have made it out to be, because there is no absolute proof that getting married will improve someone's potentially negative health outcome, and it's very important to note that unhappy marriages lead to more stress, higher blood pressures, more heart disease, more all-around health risks, and higher risk of death. One intriguing study found that women who had suffered one heart attack were more likely to suffer a second if their marriage was stressful and unhappy. (And by the way, forget that nonsense that was peddled for years for purely political reasons that men have way more to gain from marriage than women—that idea was as nutty as my trail mix because the overwhelming evidence is that good marriages provide equal measures of emotional comfort to both partners.)

- Get religion. Even as notorious an atheist as Francis Crick, the codiscoverer of the double helix, accepts that the belief in God must have some sort of biological explanation because it is so ingrained in humans. There are only two ways to explain this ubiquitous phenomenon: (1) God really does exist and She's programmed us to search for Her, or (2) for some reason, there is a God area in our brain, the original G-spot, that has persevered for eons as a protective evolutionary device, perhaps to band us together in groups for our own protection ("Hey, mess with me, mister, and my rabbi and rebitzen will get you"), or to promote better health (chanting, for example, slows heart rates, and most religions have at least some prohibitions on unhealthy activities), or (my choice) as a stress-relieving device ("I don't have to worry about that problem, dear, God will take care of it for me"). No matter the theory, though, the empirical evidence is quite convincing: people who believe in God and who join together to express that belief tend to have significantly better health outcomes than people who don't maintain religious affiliations (though I still have no idea how the researchers could distinguish between hypocrites and those with true religion). For example, in the four-decade Alameda County Study, researchers noted early on that regular churchgoers were much more likely than non-churchgoers to change their unhealthy habits to more healthful ones and to suffer less from depression. Subsequently, the researchers found that regular churchgoers, especially women, have significantly lower rates of death from cardiovascular and respiratory diseases than the nonreligious. The researchers explain these differences on the basis that churchgoers maintain healthier habits and have better social support systems, particularly more close friends and involvement in groups, than do non-churchgoers.

- Change your response to anger. Most of us hostile guys, I mean, you hostile people, do a lot of self-damage because you keep your anger pent up—you seethe—instead of blowing it off. But you can change how you handle anger, and if you do, it should provide lots of good things; in the Health Professionals Follow-Up Study, men who claimed they expressed their anger "at least some of the time" had lower risks of both heart attacks and strokes than men who never expressed their anger.

- Learn to laugh more. Laughter is, if not the best medicine for stress, then pretty close to whatever is in first place. According to a study from California, just anticipating a good laugh is enough to lead to positive, stress-lowering biological changes. In another hospital study of patients, people with heart disease were "40 percent less likely to laugh" in a variety of situations (such as when the nurses didn't get the bedpan to them quickly enough, I suppose). And in an interesting study from Japan, researchers took a handful of people out for a meal on two nights. On the first night, after the meal, the test subjects were exposed to a "boring lecture" (probably something on Japanese public radio). On the second night, the test subjects were taken out for "an evening of laughter" (probably listening to "Moon River" crooners at the local karaoke bar). The group had significantly better blood glucose levels after the laughter than they did after the speech.

- If you can't learn to laugh, then at least learn to think more highly of yourself. According to a study from San Francisco, assessing yourself as rich and powerful can help keep you healthy, which is why I've begun to insist my wife and friends call me "Hillary Clinton." So far, it hasn't worked, though.

- Learn to accept that growing old is a hell of a lot better than the alternative. Sure, you can Botox and liposuck and collagen and tint and dye your way to looking a few months younger than the geezer you'll soon become, but you know, nature is never fooled; nor is anyone else. Accept your age gracefully, because you might live longer as a result. A study that followed several hundred people for over 23 years found that those who "reported having a positive attitude toward aging lived on average more than seven years longer" than those who were more negative about facing the inevitable. That doesn't mean you shouldn't use whatever cosmetic means you like to improve your outer self. *Au contraire.* If you're going to feel more positively about yourself as a result, use any method you like to make yourself look younger. It's just that I think you're eventually going to have to accept that, well, aging is aging, and it's not so bad, and the sooner you do that, the better you'll do. But that's just me. Many of my women friends don't agree with me, but then what else is new?

- One thing I wouldn't do, though, in dealing with stress is learn to rely on herbs (or drugs) for help; even if herbs such as kava and ginseng and valerian and so on work (and that's still a big "if"), and even if they're safe (an equally big "if"), eventually, you're going to have to deal with life's issues by yourself, anyway, so why employ intermediaries in the meantime? Just because something is natural doesn't make it safe, useful, or desirable.

I will not go into detail about alternative stress relievers, but they're all worth pursuing:

- Yoga
- Relaxation therapy
- Biofeedback
- Meditation
- Cognitive behavior therapy
- Pilates
- Anything that gives you good karma and keeps the bad vibes away (yes, including dye jobs)

Om.

CHAPTER

10

Sex

Just Don't Frighten the Horses, Dear

Does it really matter what these affectionate people do—
so long as they don't do it in the streets and frighten the
horses!

MRS. PATRICK CAMPBELL

I know nothing about sex because I was always married.

ZSA ZSA GABOR

"SO THEY WANT ME to write a chapter on sex in
this new book I'm working on," I told my son
one night over dinner.

"What are they going to call it?" he asked. I should have known better than to answer him.

" 'The Good Sex Guide,' " I responded nonchalantly with the first name that popped into my head. That was, after all, the title of a TV series I'd hosted with *the* Rhona Raskin for a local channel in Vancouver, and everybody but my kids watched it (the series had lots of full frontal nudity, but my kids avoided it because they thought I was the model for those shots).

"Well," he said, "I really don't know about that."

"What do you mean?" I asked naïvely.

"I mean, if they call it 'The Good Sex Guide,' and they really want to sell copies, why would they get you to write it?"

I looked at my wife for help, but that woman just shrugged and said, "Don't look at me. I don't know why they asked you to write it, either."

When I think about it, they're right. Why did they ask me to write about sex? It's not that I can't write about sex. After all, I once penned a very sexy novel for Harlequin, but the editors rejected it as overwritten (*moi?*) and too obvious. Obvious? Well, maybe it was the title: *The Chunnel and the Train.*

But the reason I'm not sold on writing about sex is that I'm not really sure what I can tell you about good sex and lifestyle (which is my primary interest in this book) that you shouldn't already know. If you're an adult, you should have a pretty good idea of what's involved in this dance of the macabre, and if you're not an adult, then why are you reading this chapter, anyway? Put it down and go play a violent video game instead.

Indeed, when I mentioned to a British friend, radio host Philip Till, that I was going to include a section on sex in this book, he said, "Going to be a short one, isn't it, mate?" Well, yes, it is, which is probably as it should be.

You see, my main problem is that since sex is something that everyone talks about but very few people actually do something about, there are just not a lot of studies about the effects of lifestyle on sex (or of the effects of sex on health). For example, when I Googled "lifestyle and sex," I discovered that "lifestyle" is a euphemism for threesomes and swinging, which gave me no information about, say, exercise and sex, but certainly did lead me to some very interesting material (but that's stuff for another book, which I shall, of course, publish under a pseudonym). And if you look up the Sexual Health Center at *www.discovery.com*, you'll see entries for blue balls (no, thanks; as they say, been there and done that), sacred sex, and sex toys, all of which are very important issues, I'm sure, but you'll find nothing on lifestyle and sex.

That said, there are a few things to say about health and sex, and that's what follows.

Olives and Orgasms

Sex is good for you. For a start, it's good exercise. According to some experts, you can burn enough calories during sex to equal what you would expend on a good walk. Clearly, the amount of time you spend in climbing that sexual hill is an important factor in determining how many calories you actually burn during the act (or acts), but even 3 calories expended "doing it" is 3 more than you'd spend otherwise at that moment, and besides, it keeps you from migrating to the kitchen to grab another beer. So sex is good for the heart. According to Walter Willett, a famous Harvard researcher and author who addressed a conference on cancer in Oslo, Norway, the secret to a long and healthy life is Greek cuisine (I'll buy that) and lots of sex (ditto, I'm sure), or to paraphrase Walt: the secret to a long and healthy life is *olives and orgasms*. And a recent study on men backs that claim; the researchers concluded that men who ejaculated more often reported significantly better overall health than the seldom-ejaculators.

By the way, the most important part of the study actually concerned the effects on the prostate of regular "prostate exercise" (which is, of course, the only exercise many men get). The researchers concluded that "there was no association between the number of times a man ejaculated... and their... prostate size or their urine flow." In other words, it makes no difference if you do it often (alone or with company) or seldom: your prostate is an engine unto itself, guys, and will continue to grow at its own pace. Do with that information what you will, men, and soldier on.

SEX AND STRESS

Sex is also probably a good stress reducer (when it doesn't raise stress levels, that is), though I don't know of any study that has attempted to measure the stress reduction power of sex versus the stress reduction power of a placebo. I mean, it still beats me what you could use for a placebo (though I'm sure you could probably fool some guys with a beer or a bag of nachos). I also don't know of a study that has tried to compare sex with another form of stress reduction to see which works best, yet I have a sneaking suspicion that sex would not be in the top five for most people, probably not even in the top 10. For example, a British survey found that Britons are happier—

they get more of a mood lift—when they get praise from the boss, when they meet friends, or when they listen to a "special song" than when they have sex, which may tell you a lot about sex in Britain. Or not. That said, sex must certainly help lots of people sleep better, and hey, it's cheaper than relaxation therapy. Indeed, another British survey found that about 1 in 6 British women claim to use sex as a stress-relieving tool (though over 50 percent lie awake at night stressed out and too pooped to pant).

◆ ———————————————————————— ◆

Sex and Age

Age is no barrier to good sex, though the media tend to give the impression—and women's magazines certainly strongly imply—that once you're over, oh, about age 21, you don't look good enough to your partner (or to yourself) to risk getting naked in front of another human being. (I'll let the women reading this in on a little secret: no man is ever afraid of getting naked in front of anyone. In fact, the more the merrier, for most guys—"Hey, see what I got?" Why do men always think bystanders will be surprised?)

But studies continually find that sex does not necessarily get worse with age, nor do we inevitably become less attractive to our sexual partners as we grow older. Again, we turn to those sexy Brits, who did a survey on the subject of who makes the best lover. Most of the women answered that their long-term partner was "a great lover" and, for many, the best lover they had had. Sixty-five percent even claimed that sex with the right man never deteriorates, and over 50 percent thought their husband had a "gorgeous body" and nearly two-thirds still found their husband to be as attractive as when they first met. Or as the editor of the magazine that commissioned the survey said, "Truly great sex and deep intimacy are most likely to happen within... a long-term relationship."

Studies on midlife adults show that sex at midlife and beyond can be just as good as it was when you were younger (assuming it was good once), and often perhaps even better. And it's not hard to see why. For women past menopause, periods have disappeared, as the kids probably have also, so sex can be much more spontaneous, longer, more pleasurable (presumably, even the most recalcitrant male can be trained and housebroken over 15 to 20 years), and unassociated with so many of the concerns that accompany sex at a younger age. As people age, sexual activity becomes less of a "raw" experience ("Pant, pant, pant, pant. Good night. Yah, I gotta go. I'll call you. I promise.") and much more of a shared experience of emotional connection and intimacy, even for most men, who actually become better fathers, husbands, partners, and lovers as they age.

Of course, some middle-aged men do feel threatened by aging and run off with the first young Tiffany or Britney that will have them, but they are the exceptions. Most midlife men accept that their long-term relationship is, as the movie would have it, as good as it gets, and that they are in the best of possible worlds.

There is some truth to the rumor, however, that sex can get, well, a bit routine with age. Again, a British survey found that 69 percent of women said they thought of other things during sex, such as what time they would have to get up, holiday plans ("Oooh, yes, yes, yes, Ibiza!"), and, of course, home improvements ("The kitchen! The kitchen! The kitchen!").

The older you get, the more sex is also affected by other health problems you might have. Years ago, when we really didn't know much about cardiac rehabilitation, we used to tell men (it was always men, for some reason) who had suffered a heart attack to "take it easy" for many weeks, even months after the coronary event. But men being men, lots of them took that advice to its logical conclusion (to them) and they gave up on nearly all physical activities, including sex. They became what we used to call "cardiac cripples" (a term that is now politically incorrect, so no one but me uses it), men so afraid that any physical effort would produce a heart attack that they made no effort at all.

Yes, sex can kill, and a very small proportion of heart attacks do occur during sexual activity (see chapter 2), especially, it seems, if you're having an affair or a one-night stand. According to a British researcher, "75 percent of sudden death during sexual activity involved people who were taking part in extra-marital sexual intercourse." But it's an uncommon way to go even for those with significant cardiac histories, which is why doctors now encourage a vibrant sex life in cardiac patients who can manage it.

Sexual Dysfunction

One health problem associated with sex that merits special attention is ED, or what used to be known much more accurately as impotence. The reason ED merits special note is that it's intimately linked to an unhealthy lifestyle. If you have unhealthy habits—especially if you smoke and do no exercise—those arteries that feed the penis are subject to the same insults as the other arteries in your body. Because those arteries are much smaller than other arteries, they are probably even more likely to become prematurely plugged and damaged than larger arteries, such as the coronary arteries. That is why any male who is diagnosed with ED should be evaluated right away for coronary artery disease: if his willie is wilting, there's a very good chance that his heart is hobbling, too.

But a healthy lifestyle can prevent ED, and speaking as someone who exercises a lot and who has never, ever—well, I don't want to tell you more about me than you need to know. But take it from me, guys, the more active you are, the less likely you are to run into ED.

I wish I could say the same thing about sexual dysfunction in women—that a healthy lifestyle leads to less "female sexual dysfunction," a multipurpose label that has no clear definition and that covers nearly everything that prevents a woman from enjoying a good sex life. Sexual dysfunction in females is a very hot topic in medicine right now, because a number of experts have argued that we've begun to "medicalize" female sexual problems to increase the number of women who might benefit from drug therapy (drug company profits and all that) and that no one really knows what female sexual dysfunction is or even how prevalent it is. Estimates range from 43 percent of all women in one very widely cited study to a much more modest 20 to 22 percent in a more recent and, I believe, much more accurate study.

Trouble is, we know very little about lifestyle contributions to female sexual dysfunction, so all I'll say to women about lifestyle and sexual functioning is that exercising, not smoking, watching your weight, and eating well can't do your sex life any harm, and quite possibly those changes might do it a lot of good, if only because you will feel so much happier about yourself. You will probably look better, feel better, and have more energy, too.

If you don't have regular sex, then that's OK, too. Lots of people don't have sex very often, and they seem to be doing all right. A British survey found that contrary to the image you may have of the swinging young single bloke who bonks everything in sight till he drops from sheer exhaustion, 53 percent of British single men have sex only a few times a year. Fourteen percent of British married men say they have sex only a few times a year, too.

For women, a Kinsey Institute survey found that only 1 in 3 married women have sex as often as two times per week. Curiously, one of the most sexually starved groups seems to be older German women (ages 50 to 90!) a majority of whom, in a survey, told the researchers that they aren't getting enough sex because there are just not enough men around to satisfy them. But before you sell the furniture and move to Munich, let me tell you that is a common and international lament, so guys, why not stay home instead and consider pressing yourselves into local service. It's for a good cause, after all.

Finally, another British survey (for some reason, the Brits love to study their own sex lives) from a few years back found that a growing number of otherwise normally happy couples claimed to be giving up sex completely because of a loss of interest or lack of time, though these people maintained that they still loved their partners and had very good relationships. So, whatever turns you on, folks. Or not.

For those of you who want to know how to fix a poor sex life, hey, don't ask me. I suppose I could come up with a feel-good list as they do in many other medical books, with suggestions such as relax, get in the mood, dress in sexy underwear (I've tried that, by the way, but my wife hates it when I put on her bras), take time out together, use your imagination (though be warned: yogurt doesn't always work the way you'd like), build sex into your schedule ("Hey, dear, it's that time again; where are you?"), have sex in unusual places (an overweight British couple were recently named as among Britain's "worst car abusers" because they wrecked the suspension of their Mini by having bouncy, bouncy in it too often).

But, you know, I often wonder if such suggestions have ever really helped anyone improve their sex life. For me, good sex in a relationship is a two-way street (sometimes involving several lanes, of course, and even occasionally some blind curves) so if it's not working, then it's probably best to get help. Be aware, however, that many studies show that doctors may not be the best people to consult, since most doctors are too afraid or too embarrassed to discuss sex. You could, I suppose, consult a good sex manual (even if it doesn't work, the pictures are usually great), but the best way to go is probably to consult a good therapist who can work with you and your partner.

11

Issues to Discuss with Your Doctor

Mind-Melding with Your MD

Everybody wants to live forever, but nobody wants to grow old.
JONATHAN SWIFT

And one more thing ...
LT. COLUMBO, LAPD

JUST AS I WAS CELEBRATING the end of this effort with the usual glasses of bubbly, my editor was back on the phone. "Great stuff, Art," she began, and I knew right away I was in trouble. "But there's just one more thing," she added in her best Lt. Columbo voice.

"*Yessss?*" I hissed.

"Everything you wrote about can be controlled by the readers themselves. But you left out those issues you feel people need to work on with their doctor's help, such as ASA, immunizations, and especially screening tests."

"I didn't forget," I lied. "I was just thinking harder about them before submitting them."

So here they are: three final health issues that you should discuss with your doctor on your next visit.

And that's it. I promise.

ASA

Many years ago, I would have given you a clear yes-or-no answer to the question: "Should I take ASA." In those days, a doctor dispensed treatments (rarely accompanied by much useful information: "That's a pill you have to take three times a day, Mr. Bean; swallow it and have your wife call me if something goes wrong") and the grateful patient took the treatment without argument or question ("Yes, Your Grace").

But alas (that "alas" is, of course, from the perspective of a doctor who used to practice in those halcyon days), a few years ago, everything changed for reasons too confusing and bountiful to go into here, and we now have a system in which the doctor and the patient—*excuuuuse* me, the "health consumer"—are equal "partners" in decision-making, codependents in keeping the health consumer as healthy as possible. I say "as healthy as possible" because it's also well accepted in this new world that doctors don't really know much about keeping anyone completely healthy, so we settle for what we can get.

So, once I would have stated boldly that you either need to take ASA or you don't. And I would have given you doses to take and schedules to work with. And you would have been glad and thankful for a definite yes-or-no answer.

But now it's all so different, and most of you are going to have to accept the frustrating but currently chic answer that it's not at all clear what you should be doing. As a physician who suits the times—in other words, as a wishy-washy Dr. Feelgood—I can only say that I'm leaving this decision up to you and your own physician. Next.

ASA IS A NONSTEROIDAL anti-inflammatory drug, or NSAID (remember that term because it's going to come up often) that saves many lives. Unfortunately, however, studies show that many people who would benefit from regular use of ASA are simply not taking it, though on that ever-present other hand, many people who don't need ASA or for whom the benefits are not nearly as obvious are taking ASA, and therein lies the problem.

So let's review the potential benefits of ASA:

- ASA clearly lowers the risk of cardiac events, that euphemism that includes heart attacks and sudden death attributed to cardiac causes.

The Physicians' Health Study found a large 44 percent reduction in first heart attacks among doctors who used ASA, and yes, that included even doctors without major risk factors for heart disease. In a recent review of five other studies, the use of ASA in an apparently healthy population reduced the risk of a first heart attack by 32 percent and also led to a 15 percent reduction in other cardiovascular events, such as blood clots.

- ASA may prevent further cardiac damage when taken during the first signs of a heart attack. According to most health authorities, if you think you are suffering a heart attack, the first thing you ought to do is pop an ASA. And if you can think clearly, try to chew it rather than swallow it—the ASA hits the bloodstream faster when the tablet is chewed. Then call 9-1-1, and make bloody sure it's 9-1-1 and not Aunt Mathilda or your spouse that you ring in those crucial moments. Get to the hospital first and then ask your spouse or relations if that was a wise thing to do, because the sooner the doctors can get potent clot-busters into you, the better your prognosis.

ASA prevents cardiac events because it:

- Slows clotting by making platelets—those blood cells that are crucially involved in clots—less "sticky."
- Has an anti-inflammatory effect, which manifests itself both locally in the cardiac blood vessels and systemically, that is, all over the body, and you remember how important a role inflammation is thought to play in cardiac disease.
- May also have the current catch-all of an "antioxidant" effect (see chapter 3).
- Might even lower blood pressure, though according to one study, ASA can do that only if it's taken at night, not during the daytime.

Besides its potential positive effects on cardiovascular disease, ASA has other benefits as:

- A potent anti-inflammatory (ASA is very useful in the treatment of all inflammatory conditions, such as athletic injuries and arthritis).

- A fever reducer.
- A good pain reliever.

And perhaps most intriguing, ASA might have a host of other potential benefits, most probably to do with that anti-inflammatory effect. Thus, ASA might help reduce the risks of:

- *Breast cancer.* In the Women's Health Initiative Study, post-menopausal women who took regular doses of ASA had more than a 25 percent lower risk of breast cancer.
- *Colorectal cancer.* In several studies, people who were on ASA ended up with up to a 40 percent lower risk of colon cancer. In another very hyped study that was terminated early because the results were declared to be so clear and important, people at high-risk for colon polyps (precursors to colon cancer) had significantly fewer polyps when they were put on regular doses of ASA.
- *Lung cancer.* In women who are heavy smokers, ASA may lower the risk of lung cancer by about half.
- *Esophageal cancer.* According to a review of major studies, researchers determined that ASA (and other NSAIDs) lower the risk of esophageal cancer by up to 43 percent.
- *Mouth and throat cancer.* An Italian study concluded that regular low doses of ASA are associated with lower risks of cancers of the mouth and throat (as well as the esophagus).
- *Pancreatic cancer.* An American study found a lower risk of pancreatic cancer among ASA users.
- *Prostate cancer.* Men older than 60 who used daily NSAIDs were about half as likely to get prostate cancer as were nonusers of ASA.
- *Ovarian cancer.* One American study hinted at the possibility that regular use of ASA reduces the risk of one type of ovarian cancer.
- *Uterine cancer.* In the laboratory, ASA was found to inhibit the growth of uterine cancer cells.

So that's ASA's impressive potential anticancer effect. On top of that, there's even the intriguing prospect that ASA might reduce the risk of Alzheimer's disease. A study from Mormon country found that people who had taken regular doses of ASA (or other NSAIDs) for at least two years were less likely to end up with Alzheimer's disease and other forms of dementia than nonusers of ASA. Starting to take ASA once Alzheimer's had set in did not provide any relief from the disease, however.

In summary, ASA might reduce the risk of:

- Heart attack
- Some kinds of stroke
- Blood clots
- Alzheimer's disease
- Breast cancer
- Lung cancer
- Colorectal cancer
- Esophageal cancer
- A host of other cancers

So if it can do all that, why shouldn't everybody take ASA? The problem is that there are a number of drawbacks and potential hazards associated with its use. ASA:

- Increases the risk of that type of stroke known as a hemorrhagic stroke, which is due to bleeding in the brain. This drawback is directly related to one of the major positive effects of ASA, namely it's ability to slow clotting.
- Increases the risk of bleeding from the stomach, which not only may lead to anemia but also interferes with the accuracy of some screening tests for colon cancer.
- Increases the risk of sudden rupture of a stomach ulcer. This potentially life-threatening complication can often come on with no pre-existing symptoms, and is not reduced by taking "coated" ASA. Also, the longer you take ASA, the higher your risk of suffering such a bleed; one review in the *British Medical Journal* put it like this: "Long term therapy with [ASA] is associated with a *significant* [emphasis added] increase in gastrointestinal hemorrhage. No evidence exists that reducing the dose or using modified formulations would reduce the incidence of gastrointestinal hemorrhage."

- Increases "gastritis" symptoms, such as burning and indigestion.
- May worsen chronic heart failure.
- Leads to asthma and allergic symptoms.
- Interacts with other medications.
- May become more of a problem the older we get, meaning that GI hemorrhages (and perhaps heart failure), as complications of using ASA, become more likely as we age.

Finally, and this is very important, no one really knows the dose that should be used for any of these benefits, even for the prevention of heart problems. Sure, your doctor might tell you, with a definitive tone and manner, to take a whole ASA (325 mg) a day or a "baby" ASA (81 mg) daily, or half an ASA every second day. But he's guessing at all these doses.

As for the potential benefits against cancer or Alzheimer's disease, again, the dose is all over the map. In the Women's Health Initiative, the anti-breast-cancer benefit was found only for regular ASA doses, not for baby ASA. Just to drive you crazy, a much touted study published in the *New England Journal of Medicine* found that ASA reduced the risk of getting precancerous polyps in the bowel but that the only dose that worked was the baby dose. The full dose of ASA didn't reduce the risk of polyps. Why would a small dose of ASA help prevent cancer, whereas a larger dose wouldn't?

If you want to win a big prize, 'splain that, if you can, Lucy.

The fact is no one knows the right dose to give the best protection while offering the minimum risk. That said, the consensus seems to be that one baby ASA a day offers adequate cardiac protection for most people, but whether that also offers protection against other health problems remains to be determined.

Also—and this is becoming apparent as more and more people are self-medicating with ASA—some people are "resistant" to the effects of ASA, so they really have nothing to gain from using it and everything to lose. How can you tell if you are resistant? Sorry, but without specialized tests, you can't.

Finally, some evidence points to the fact that taking other anti-inflammatories, such as ibuprofen, for chronic pain or arthritis, say, might even negate some of the positive effects of ASA.

So, putting all that together, who should be on ASA?

- Nearly everyone with a previous heart attack or ischemic stroke (stroke caused by a clot in a blood vessel to the brain) can benefit from using ASA.
- People at high risk for heart attack, especially those with diabetes, and probably, too, those with the metabolic syndrome, the obese, those with a family history of premature heart disease, smokers, and those with elevated cholesterol levels generally also have more to gain than to lose from taking ASA.

The kind folks at the American Heart Association (AHA) have come up with the following guidelines (it's on their Web site, which is definitely worth a visit): ASA should be used by people who have a risk of 10 percent or more of suffering a heart attack over the next 10 years. Even this is somewhat disputed, though, because some doctors believe that anyone with a risk of 6 percent or more over the next 10 years should probably take ASA. And remember, that's only if you're worried about cardiac risks. The AHA is not interested in your breast cancer risks or the risks to your tush.

Those of us at average or low risk for cardiac events—your baby-boomer male or female who works out, eats well, and doesn't smoke—should probably not take ASA regularly, though clearly many are. According to data from the 20-year Minnesota Heart Study, 52 percent of low-risk (for cardiac needs) men and 31 percent of low-risk women are taking ASA regularly.

Why are they doing that? Because most people don't know how to evaluate their own cardiac risk, and since nearly everyone views ASA as a completely risk-free drug, they figure that there's no harm in it, so why not take it, eh?

I urge you to be cautious about doing that, though. I may be a lonely voice and this may be an unpopular view, but I believe the benefits of ASA have been hyped and the drawbacks largely ignored, much as with HRT, and that worries me.

Finally, those who should be very cautious about their use of ASA include people:

- With a bleeding disorder.
- Allergic to ASA.
- On another drug that has similar actions to ASA, such as one of the other nonsteroidal anti-inflammatory drugs.
- With heart failure. An American study found that NSAIDs can increase the risk of heart failure by up to 60 percent.
- With kidney disease.

So there you have it. As I said, it's up to you now, pardner.

Tests and Immunizations

Hey, know what? I even managed to practice method writing in this section; to wit, I got my lipid levels done and I got my second hepatitis A shot. And it still hurts. Just kidding. It didn't hurt in the least, though I took no chances and had my daily two glasses of Shiraz just before getting the shot. Never even noticed the needle going in.

EXAMINATIONS

Let's start with what you need to get checked out periodically in your doctor's office. I assume that if you have a specific health complaint—a lump, a previous cancer—or if you are on medication, that you are smart enough to have discussed with your doctor how often you should see her. If you are not that smart, make sure you see your doctor soon to discuss your monitoring schedule.

Blood pressure

You should get your blood pressure checked routinely when you visit a doctor's office, and if you're fortunate enough not to have to visit the doctor, then you should get your blood pressure checked every two years, anyway. If your blood pressure is generally normal and you haven't had major changes in your life, you can get it measured at the local pharmacy or even at your local supermarket, but bear in mind that those machines are not as accurate as your doctor's blood pressure machine (I hate to tell you how inaccurate even your doctor's blood pressure machine may be, so I won't).

A very important caution: never accept either one or two abnormal blood readings as a sure sign that you have high blood pressure. If your

blood pressure is abnormal, always get at least three readings on separate occasions several weeks apart before accepting that it really is high.
(There is even some controversy as to whether blood pressure readings
are more accurate early in the day or later in the afternoon, but let's not
go there for now.) And always make sure you know the exact numbers,
OK? If you can remember your phone number, you can remember your
blood pressure, and if you can't remember your phone number, then
don't worry about your blood pressure. It's the least of your problems.

Breast exam in women

Although I can find little evidence that annual breast examination by a
clinician (or regular breast self-examination) saves lives, everyone recommends that women get regular breast exams from a health professional and I am not about to swim against that tide, especially since I'm
such a poor swimmer. At the very least, the need for an annual breast
examination brings lots of women into the doctor's office, where they
can discuss other important health issues that might save their lives.

Pelvic examination

This is a tough one to deal with because women hate it and it's hard to
come up with data to justify doing it routinely (the Pap smear is a separate issue—see below). In a pelvic examination, the ovaries and lower
abdomen are palpated, and often a digital rectal examination is included just for good measure to check for rectal cancer and ovarian
cancer. An ovarian cancer, though, is not easy to palpate when it's
small enough to be easily treated (which is part of the reason ovarian
cancer has a poor prognosis, not to mention that one study found that
ovarian cancer symptoms are often ignored for months as being "too
vague" by both the doctor and the patient). On top of that, according to
a recent study, unless your doctor has longer than average digits, she's
unlikely to pick up most rectal cancers. (But then do you really want a
doctor with digits as long as a hockey stick? I think not.)

Again, lots of experts recommend pelvic examination on a routine
basis, so I'm not about to say don't do it. But do talk it over with your
doctor before blindly rushing in to get yours done this year.

Rectal examination

As with breast examination, I am not at all convinced that a good case can be made that routine digital rectal examinations (the dreaded DRE) save lives. As noted above, a great many rectal cancers are not palpable on DRE, and many prostate cancers have metastasized by the time they can be palpated on rectal examination. Moreover, most prostate "lumps" felt on DRE do not turn out to be cancer, yet all such lumps have to be investigated further, often with surgical biopsy, leading to needless worry, expense, and worst of all, risk of complications. But again, I feel it's urgent to get elderly gents into the office to discuss important health matters, and if this is the only way to do that, well, so be it.

While we're down in that area, one examination that actually does save lives is testicular self-examination, especially in young men, so every young boy should be taught to roll his own.

Skin examination

Your skin should be examined periodically for suspicious-looking spots. In low-risk individuals this doesn't have to be done by a health professional; your partner could do it for you, turning it into a very fun procedure.

Eye examination

You should get your eyes checked from time to time because as you get older, two problems—glaucoma and age-related maculopathy—become more common without necessarily producing much in the way of symptoms. Trouble is, most family doctors don't check for these conditions adequately, so yes, see an eye specialist from time to time.

AND THAT'S ALL she wrote, folks. No, you don't need an annual physical exam, since no study has ever shown that annual physical exams save lives, though they do make both patients and doctors feel better— patients because they think that when they get a clean bill of health following an examination they're actually healthy (it means no such thing) and doctors because a physical exam makes them feel useful, and besides, full physicals are so lucrative.

SCREENING TESTS

Lipid profile

I encourage every adult (and probably every kid) to learn their lipid profile, though I know that most of you won't do much about it even if your lipid levels are atrocious. But even if just a few of you pay more attention to your health as a result of such a test, then my work will have been worth it because you may put off your assignation with the Angel of Death. As a doctor, I know one thing for sure: everyone, including Her, can be made to wait in the waiting room.

How often should your lipid profile be repeated? Probably every five years, if it's normal, in men and postmenopausal women.

Blood glucose

Current consensus recommendations are to get a glucose test for diabetes at age 45, and then routinely (every two to three years) after that. But since more people are fatter at an earlier age now—and hence at a hugely increased risk of diabetes—glucose screening is probably warranted for younger people when they have significant risk factors such as obesity or a strong family history of diabetes (as well as for women who deliver big babies).

Thyroid hormone

Ten percent of women over the age of 50 are hypothyroid (meaning the thyroid hormone level is too low), leaving them at higher risk of all sorts of health problems, including a higher risk of heart disease. So, I asks you, folks, don't it make sense that all women of that certain age check their thyroid status periodically? Yes, it do.

CRP and homocysteine levels

Boy, oh boy, are these two ever hot potatoes! I think that both are going to become routine tests in the next five years in the U.S. (10 years in much slower Canada), but for now, they are rarely done, and the authorities are begging us not to use the tests widely until we know more about them. That said, I think that anyone with an added risk for heart disease—family history of premature heart disease, high blood pressure, diabetes—should get these checked out. A great place to get more information about this test—and all similar heart-related tests, as well as a cardiac risk assessment—is at the American Heart Association Web site, *americanheart.com*—(and no, you don't have to have an American heart to access the site).

In the list of screening tests that are not blood tests, the only ones I can recommend are those that follow.

STD *testing*
The tests required here vary tremendously according to risk, but all women who are sexually active should probably be screened for chlamydia.

Bone density test
Every woman should have bone density tests starting at around age 50 (sooner if menopause was early). Twenty percent of women who suffer a hip fracture die, and a further 25 percent never recover their mobility. Most didn't even know they had thin bones and so weren't encouraged to do much to prevent this awful complication. And bone thinning starts much sooner than you think. A recent study of over 90,000 women found that nearly a third of women between the ages of 50 and 64—relatively young women, in other words—already had a low enough bone mass to put them at three times the normal risk of fracture. In fact, 20 percent of hip fractures in this study occurred in women under the age of 65.

Osteoporosis affects men, too. About 30 percent of men over the age of 65 have osteoporosis, about a third of all hip fractures occur in men, and men tend to do much worse after they fracture a hip than do women. So this recommendation also applies to my elderly brothers: get your bones evaluated.

ECG
I don't believe in routine ECGs, but I do believe that a stress ECG (done while you are working out on a treadmill) should be done on any previously sedentary middle-aged adult who starts a new exercise program and on anyone with increased risk of dying suddenly during exercise. If they ever figure out how to do this one more cheaply and with fewer personnel, I will recommend that everyone get it.

CT scans

Here's yet another very controversial test: CT scans (computerized X rays) pick up heart disease by detecting calcium build-up in the coronary arteries (the official name for the test is electron beam computed tomography, or EBCT). The controversy does not stem from the effectiveness of these tests, because I think everyone agrees that EBCT does pick up calcium deposits, and it can do that in otherwise healthy individuals with seemingly no risk for heart disease (remember that half of all heart attacks occur in people with presumably normal lipid levels and without previous symptoms of heart disease). The problems with EBCT are:

- It's expensive.
- It involves extra radiation (albeit small amounts).
- EBCT is so new that no study has yet shown that people who have been diagnosed with premature heart disease simply on the basis of EBCT live any longer as a result of finding out the state of their arteries.
- CT scans can engender lots of anxiety (many people who go for them have had no inkling that they might have any heart problems), but so can any other screening test.

Should you get one? Well, I did, but I'm not you. You? I have no idea. Remember that this is a new era. Your call, I'm afraid.

On to screening cancer checks, and this is probably the most controversial list of all.

Mammograms

Annual or biannual mammograms do save lives in older women and should probably start at age 40, but at the latest age 50. I am not nearly as sure, however, that putting a 75-year-old woman through the hassle of routine mammography, with its high risk of false positive readings— 10 percent of mammograms show "something" that must be followed up but that turns out to be "nothing"—is worth the little bit of benefit a woman of that age might gain from the slightly earlier detection of a breast cancer that is not likely to kill her, anyway. But hey, that's only me. The experts say that if a woman has a good 10 years of life left, then she should be screened routinely with mammograms, no matter how old she is.

By the way, for those women who've put off getting a mammogram because they've heard that mammograms hurt too much (for men who wonder how a measly little X ray could possibly hurt, the equivalent procedure would be to have your balls placed on an ice-cold tray and squeezed between two metal plates while an attendant stands in the other room and yells, "Don't breathe"), a recent study found that most women say the pain of a mammogram is not nearly as bad as they thought it would be, and very few women say that the pain would preclude them from getting another mammogram in the future.

Pap smears
This test for cervical cancer is absolutely necessary and clearly saves lives, though the frequency depends on your risk profile. Be sure to discuss yours with your doctor.

Colon cancer
Colorectal cancer is the second leading cause of cancer death in North America, even though it is very preventable if caught early, in the pre-malignant polyp stage, so this is a very valuable screening test. Unfortunately it is not used much and is even more poorly administered and followed up on, in large part because we live in a world that's got a taboo on poo-poo. In fact, many more men seem to get the PSA test for prostate cancer (see below) than colon cancer screening, though the PSA test has not established its worth to nearly the same extent. One study found that only 50 percent of people over 50 have had even one colon cancer screening test. So I don't care if you choose:

- A stool test for occult blood, in which you have to (yuck!) collect one to three stool samples—yes, with a little stick, thank God—and smear them on a special card that you then deliver, gingerly, to the lab or doctor's office (once a year).
- A colonoscopy (best), in which a scope is navigated all the way through the colon (every 10 years, and that's mostly why it's best).

Just pick your method and get it done routinely. And if you have a positive test, make sure it's followed up appropriately! This one saves lives. And even as you read this, colon cancer researchers are avidly pursuing improvements on this test, such as blood tests and genetic fingerprinting (don't ask).

Prostate specific antigen (PSA)

This is the very controversial blood test for prostate cancer. I believe it works to reduce death from prostate cancer, and I would advise every man over 50 to get it (African-American men over age 40). Depending on the PSA level, you should then get the test either every year or every two years. In men with a strong family history of prostate cancer (fathers, brothers, even granddad or a cousin), it should be done annually from the age of 40.

An important caution: a recent study showed that PSA levels can vary quite a bit, depending on several factors, including even when they're taken. So if you have a mildly elevated PSA level, before allowing yourself to endure a prostate biopsy to search for cancer, always ask to have the test repeated first, a few weeks later. There's a good chance your level will have returned to normal, and you will then thank the Lord that you bought this book.

IMMUNIZATIONS

Vaccines that many of you should either get *de novo* or update include those for:

- Pneumococcal disease
- Hepatitis B
- Hepatitis A
- Mumps, measles, and rubella
- Diphtheria and tetanus
- Whooping cough
- Polio
- Meningitis
- Flu virus (which is the only one I will discuss in detail because it can save so many lives)

Traditionally, flu shots have been recommended for:

- Health care workers.
- Anyone with a chronic health condition such as asthma, kidney disease, diabetes, or heart disease.
- People over the age of 65.
- Residents of nursing homes and long-term care facilities.
- People with a compromised immune system such as those with HIV/AIDS, people on immune suppressant drugs, or people without a spleen.
- Those who take care of people with chronic illness or who are likely to transmit flu to high-risk individuals.
- Women in the second or third trimester of their pregnancies.

But that was then and this is now. Now we know that nearly everyone would benefit from an annual flu shot. American authorities recommend flu shots for healthy kids over the age of two as well as for all adults over the age of 50.

Does that mean that people between the ages of 16 and 49 don't need a flu shot? Not at all. It's just that there's not enough flu vaccine to go around for everyone, so some restrictions are necessary. But most immunization experts counsel that if you want a flu shot, you should get one, no matter what your age.

What does a flu shot do? Two things: (1) it reduces the risks of getting the flu by anywhere from 70 to 80 percent, and (2) even if you get the flu, a flu shot significantly cuts your chances of getting complications such as pneumonia. And if you don't think that's a big deal, think again. People who get flu shots:

- Have lower risks of dying of any cause. A study of over 100,000 Swedish seniors found that the overall risk of death was cut by 57 percent in those immunized against the flu and pneumonia (see below).
- Spend much less time in hospital. That same Swedish study also found that flu immunization cut the risk of hospitalization by 46 percent.

- Have a lower risk of heart attack and stroke. In Minnesota, flu vaccination of the elderly was found to cut the stroke risk by 23 percent and hospitalization for heart disease by 19 percent.
- Lose much less time from work.
- Spend much less on anti-flu medications.

Why do you need an annual flu shot? Because the flu virus is like a kid you send off to college—it mutates quickly. So every year, there's a slightly different version of the flu virus out there causing all those sniffles, coughs, and general aches, and the shot you got last year won't protect you against the new version doing the rounds.

Are there any drawbacks to getting a flu shot? Yes:

- It may not work.
- It causes a slight ache in the arm.
- Occasionally it causes reactions (such as runny eyes and mild congestion).

One thing the flu shot does not do is cause the flu. Why, then, do so many people complain that "last year, you talked me into that damn flu shot, Doc, and then I got the sickest I've been in years"? Because after they get a flu shot, many people naturally blame the shot for everything bad that happens to them subsequently.

Another thing the flu shot does not do is lower your immunity so that you won't be able to fight off future flu infections. There is absolutely no evidence that immunizations negatively impact immunity.

And, oh yes, when you go for your annual flu shot this year—you will go, won't you?—try to be as relaxed and well rested as you can be. Studies show that high stress levels and lack of sleep both lower the effectiveness of flu vaccination.

Conclusion

All Good Things Must Come to an End

I don't know why we are here, but I'm pretty sure that it is not in order to enjoy ourselves.
LUDWIG WITTGENSTEIN

In theory, there is no difference between theory and practice. But, in practice, there is.
JAN L.A. VAN DE SNEPSCHEUT

So, THERE YOU HAVE IT, folks: a compendium of my knowledge about what makes for a longer and healthier life. But just because so many of my readers are in midlife or beyond, I think it's best if I briefly restate some of the more important elements of a lifestyle geared to helping you living longer:

- Exercise for at least one half-hour most days of the week.
- Eat a varied and healthy diet, focusing on fruits and veggies, legumes, fish, whole grains, and monounsaturated fats (to replace saturated fats and especially trans fats).
- Watch your portions but don't skip meals, and snack if you feel hungry.
- Drink wine in moderate amounts (though if you don't drink alcohol, I am not about to tell you to start now).

- Stop smoking.
- Get enough sleep to be well-rested the next day.
- Develop strategies to minimize the effects of the inevitable stresses we all face on a regular basis.

And that's all she wrote, folks. Yes, your mother could have told you the same things, but you must admit that she would never have put it as nicely as I did. Or had the studies to back up what she said.

This entire effort, by the way, was predicated on two simple premises: (1) that I do not have a monopoly on information that will allow you to live a healthier life, and (2) that unlike that party animal, Ludwig Wittgenstein, you actually want to enjoy your life while improving your chances of living longer. So if and when you make some of the changes I've suggested, bear both those caveats in mind at all times. Other people will undoubtedly offer you different advice, and they may be just as right as I am—perhaps even more right (*Nahh!* How could that be?)—because unlike George Bernard Shaw, who said, "The longer I live the more I see that I am never wrong about anything," I accept that I am not always right and that what I say is often not the last word. Hey, constantly being reminded of that is what's gotten me through 33 years of happy marriage.

Besides, some study I authoritatively cite today may be totally contradicted tomorrow, and today's prevalent theory may be tomorrow's equivalent of fish wrap.

So by all means, consult other sources, and if you prefer to believe someone other than me, hey, I'm a big boy, and I can handle it. In the end, all I want is for you to make the best choices possible for yourself, and choices that will lead to more—not less—enjoyment of life.

Let me close by offering this final message: healthy living is like sex (what isn't?)—if you put in the time and the effort, the payoff can be stupendous. If you don't put in that effort, well, the sex may be good, anyway—after all, there are no bad orgasms, I believe—but it won't be nearly as good as if you had worked at it, though you may never know that if you don't do the work.

Ah, well, time now to heed my own advice. First, some extraordinary olives, and then ... well, if the missus is home, a long walk, of course. Or whatever.

Bibliography

GENERAL

Atkins, Robert C., M.D. *Dr. Atkins' New Diet Revolution.* New York: Avon Books, 1999.

Balch, James F., M.D., and Phyllis A. Balch, C.N.C. *Prescription for Nutritional Healing: A Practical A–Z Reference to Drug-Free Remedies Using Vitamins, Minerals, Herbs, and Food Supplements.* Garden City: Avery Publishing Group, 1990.

Banks, Ian, M.D. *Ask Dr. Ian about Sex.* Belfast: Blackstaff Press, 1999.

Benson, Herbert, M.D., Ellen M. Stuart, R.N., M.S. and the Staff of the Mind/Body Medical Institute of New England Deaconess Hospital and Harvard Medical School. *The Wellness Book: The Comprehensive Guide to Maintaining Health and Treating Stress-Related Illness.* New York: Birch Lane Press, 1992

Caldwell, J. Paul. *Sleep.* Toronto: Key Porter Books, 1995.

Inlander, Charles B. and the Staff of the People's Medical Society. *People's Medical Society Men's Health and Wellness Encyclopedia.* New York: Macmillan, 1998.

Kolata, Gina. *Ultimate Fitness: The Quest for Truth About Health and Exercise.* New York: Farrar, Straus and Giroux, 2003.

Mate, Gabor, M.D. *When the Body Says No: The Cost of Hidden Stress.* Toronto: Alfred A. Knopf Canada, 2003.

Ornish, Dean, M.D. *Dr. Dean Ornish's Program for Reversing Heart Disease.* New York: Ivy Books, 1996.

Shils, Maurice E., James A. Olson, Moshe Shike, and A. Catharine Ross, eds. *Modern Nutrition in Health and Disease.* Philadelphia: Lea and Feibiger, 1994.

Vaillant, George E. M.D. *Aging Well: Surprising Guideposts to a Happier Life from the Landmark Harvard Study of Adult Development.* Boston: Little, Brown, 2002.

Weil, Andrew, M.D. *Eating Well for Optimum Health: The Essential Guide to Bringing Health and Pleasure Back to Eating.* New York: HarperCollins, 2001.

Weil, Andrew, M.D. *Eight Weeks to Optimum Health: A Proven Program for Taking Full Advantage of Your Body's Natural Healing Power.* New York: Fawcett Columbine, 1998.

Willcox, Bradley J., M.D., Craig Willcox, PhD., and Makoto Suzuki, M.D. *The Okinawa Program: How the World's Longest-Lived People Achieve Everlasting Health—and How You Can Too.* New York: Three Rivers Press, 2001.

Willett, Walter. *Eat, Drink, and Be Healthy: The Harvard Medical School Guide to Healthy Eating.* New York: Simon and Schuster, 2001.

CHAPTERS 1 AND 2: EXERCISE AND GETTING STARTED

Blackman, M.R., et al. "Growth Hormone and Sex Steroid Administration in Healthy Aged Women and Men: A Randomized Controlled Trial." *Journal of the American Medical Association* 288 (2002): 2282–92.

Blair S.N., and S. Brodney. "Effects of Physical Inactivity and Obesity on Morbidity and Mortality: Current Evidence and Research Issues." *Medicine and Science in Sports and Exercise* 31, suppl. (1999): S646–S662.

Blair, S.N., et al. "Influences of Cardiorespiratory Fitness and Other Precursors on Cardiovascular Disease and All-Cause Mortality in Men and Women." *Journal of the American Medical Association* 276 (1996): 205–10.

Centers for Disease Control and Prevention, and National Center for Chronic Disease Prevention and Promotion. *Physical Activity and Health: A Report of the Surgeon General.* Atlanta, GA: U.S. Department of Health and Human Services, 1996.

Goldbourt U., et al. "Isolated Low HDL Cholesterol as a Risk Factor for Coronary Heart Disease Mortality: A 21-Year Follow-Up of 8,000 Men." *Arteriosclerosis, Thrombosis, and Vascular Biology* 17 (1997): 107–13.

Hakim, A.A., et al. "Effects of Walking on Mortality Among Nonsmoking Retired Men." *New England Journal of Medicine* 338 (1998): 94–99.

Knowler W.C., et al. "Reduction in the Incidence of Type 2 Diabetes with Lifestyle Intervention or Metformin." *New England Journal of Medicine* 346 (2002): 393–403.

Kujala, V.M., et al. "Relationship of Leisure-Time Physical Activity and Mortality: The Finnish Twin Cohort." *Journal of the American Medical Association* 279 (1998): 440–44.

Kushi L.H., et al. "Physical Activity and Mortality in Postmenopausal Women." *Journal of the American Medical Association* 277 (1997): 1287–92.

Lee I.M., et al. "Exercise Intensity and Longevity in Men. The Harvard Alumni Health Study." *Journal of the American Medical Association* 273 (1995): 1179–84.

McGuire D.K., et al. "A 30-Year Follow-Up of the Dallas Bed Rest and Training Study: I. Effect of Age on the Cardiovascular Response to Exercise." *Circulation* 104 (2001): 1350–57.

McGuire D.K., et al. "A 30-Year Follow-Up of the Dallas Bed Rest and Training Study: II. Effect of Age on Cardiovascular Adaptation to Exercise Training." *Circulation* 104 (2001): 1358–66.

Mittleman, M.A., et al. for the Determinants of Myocardial Infarction Onset Study Investigators. "Triggering of Acute Myocardial Infarction by Heavy Physical Exertion—Protection Against Triggering by Regular Exertion." *New England Journal of Medicine* 329 (1993): 1677–83.

Nygard, O., et al. "Plasma Homocysteine Levels and Mortality in Patients with Coronary Artery Disease." *New England Journal of Medicine* 337 (1997): 230–36.

Paffenberger, R.S., et al. "The Association of Changes in Physical Activity Level and Other Lifestyle Characteristics with Mortality Among Men." *New England Journal of Medicine* 328 (1993): 538–45.

Pearson, T., et al. "Markers of Inflammation and Cardiovascular Disease: Application to Clinical and Public Health Practice—A Statement for Health Care Professionals from the Centers of Disease Control and Prevention and the American Heart Association." *Circulation* 107 (2003): 499–511.

Pouliot, M.C., et al. "Visceral Obesity in Men: Associations with Glucose Tolerance, Plasma Insulin, and Lipoprotein Levels." *Diabetes* 41 (1992): 826–34.

Rexrode, K.M., et al. "Abdominal Adiposity and Coronary Heart Disease in Women." *Journal of the American Medical Association* 280 (1998): 1843–48.

Ross, R. "Atherosclerosis—An Inflammatory Disease." *New England Journal of Medicine* 340 (1999): 115–26.

Rudman, D. "Effects of Human Growth Hormone in Men over 60 Years Old." *New England Journal of Medicine.* 323 (1990): 1–5.

Systolic Hypertension in the Elderly Program (SHEP). "Effect of Treating Isolated Systolic Hypertension on the Risk of Developing Various Types and Subtypes of Stroke." *Journal of the American Medical Association* 284 (2000): 465–71.

Van der Hoogen, P.C., et al. "The Relation Between Blood Pressure and Mortality Due to Coronary Heart Disease Among Men in Different Parts of the World." *New England Journal of Medicine* 342 (2000): 1–8.

Vance, M.L. "Can Growth Hormone Prevent Aging?" *New England Journal of Medicine.* 348 (2003): 779–80.

Wannamethee, S.G., et al. "Changes in Physical Activity, Mortality and Incidence of Coronary Heart Disease in Older Men." *The Lancet* 351 (1998): 1603–8.

Williams, P.T. "Relationships of Heart Disease Risk Factors to Exercise Quantity and Intensity." *Archives of Internal Medicine* 158 (1998): 237–45.

CHAPTERS 3 AND 4: EATING PROPERLY AND NUTRITION

Albert, C.M., et al. "Fish Consumption and Risk of Sudden Cardiac Death." *Journal of the American Medical Association* 279 (1998): 23–28.

Alberts, D.S., et al. "Lack of Effect of a High-Fiber Cereal Supplement on the Recurrence of Colorectal Adenomas." *New England Journal of Medicine* 342 (2000): 1156–1162.

Alpha-Tocopherol Beta-Carotene Cancer Prevention Study Group. "The Effect of Vitamin E and Beta-Carotene on the Incidence of Lung Cancer and Other Cancers in Male Smokers." *New England Journal of Medicine* 330 (1994): 1029.

Anderson, J.W. "Meta-Analysis of the Effects of Soy Protein Intake on Serum Lipids." *New England Journal of Medicine* 333 (1995): 276–82.

Antonios, T.F.T., and G.A. MacGregor. "Salt: More Adverse Effects." *The Lancet* 348 (1996): 250–51.

Appel, L.J., et al., for the DASH Collaborative Research Group. "A Clinical Trial of the Effects of Dietary Patterns on Blood Pressure." *New England Journal of Medicine* 336 (1997): 1117–24.

Ascherio, A., et al. "Dietary Intake of Marine N-3 Fatty Acids, Fish Intake, and the Risk of Coronary Disease Among Men." *New England Journal of Medicine* 332 (1995): 977–82.

Ascherio, A., et al. "A Prospective Study of Nutritional Factors and Hypertension Among U.S. Men." *Circulation* 86 (1992): 1475–84.

Ascherio, A., et al. "Trans Fatty Acids and Coronary Heart Disease." *New England Journal of Medicine* 340 (1999): 1994–98.

Bazzano, L.A., et al. "Dietary Intake of Folate and Risk of Stroke in U.S. Men and Women: NHANES I Epidemiologic Follow-Up Study." *Stroke* 33 (2002): 1183–89.

Bronstrup, A., et al. "Effects of Folic Acid and Combinations of Folic Acid and Vitamin B12 on Plasma Homocysteine Concentrations in Healthy, Young Women." *American Journal of Clinical Nutrition* 68 (1998): 1104–10.

Brown, L., et al. "Cholesterol-Lowering Effects of Dietary Fiber: A Meta-Analysis." *American Journal of Clinical Nutrition* 69 (1999): 30–42.

Brunner, E., et al. "Can Dietary Interventions Change Diet and Cardiovascular Risk Factors? A Meta-Analysis of Randomized Controlled Trials." *American Journal of Public Health* 87 (1997): 1415–22.

Christen, W.G., et al. "Design of Physicians' Health Study II—A Randomized Trial of Beta-Carotene, Vitamins E and C, and Multivitamins, in Prevention of Cancer, Cardiovascular Disease, and Eye Disease, and Review of Results of Completed Trials." *Annals of Epidemiology* 10 (2000): 125.

Compston, J.E. "Vitamin D Deficiency: Time for Action: Evidence Supports Routine Supplementation for Elderly People and Others at Risk." *British Medical Journal* 317 (1998): 1466–67.

Cutler, J.A., et al. "Randomized Trials of Sodium Reduction: An Overview." *American Journal of Clinical Nutrition* 65, suppl. (1997): 643S–651S.

Daviglus, M.L., et al. "Fish Consumption and the 30-Year Risk of Fatal Myocardial Infarction." *New England Journal of Medicine* 336 (1997): 1046–53.

Dawson-Hughes, B., et al. "Effect of Calcium and Vitamin D Supplementation on Bone Density in Men and Women 65 Years of Age or Older." *New England Journal of Medicine* 337 (1997): 670–76.

De Lorgeril, M., et al. "Mediterranean Alpha-Linoleic Acid-Rich Diet in Secondary Prevention of Coronary Heart Disease." *The Lancet* 343 (1994): 1454–59.

Diaz, M.N., et al. "Antioxidants and Atherosclerotic Heart Disease." *New England Journal of Medicine* 337 (1997): 408.

Erdman, J.W. AHA Science Advisory: Soy Protein and Cardiovascular Disease: A Statement for Healthcare Professionals from the Nutrition Committee of the AHA." *Circulation.* 102 (2000): 2555–59.

Ernst, N.D., et al. "Consistency between U.S. Dietary Fat Intake and Serum Total Cholesterol Concentrations: The National Health and Nutrition Examination Surveys." *American Journal of Clinical Nutrition* 66, suppl. (1997): 965S–972S.

Foley, M., et al. "Should Mono- or Poly-Unsaturated Fats Replace Saturated Fat in the Diet?" *European Journal of Clinical Nutrition* 46 (1992): 429–36.

Fuchs, C.S., et al. "Dietary Fiber and the Risk of Colorectal Cancer and Adenoma in Women." *New England Journal of Medicine* 340 (1999): 169–76.

Gardner, C.D., and H.C. Kraemer, "Monounsaturated Versus Polyunsaturated Dietary Fat and Serum Lipids: A Meta-Analysis." *Arteriosclerosis, Thrombosis, and Vascular Biology* 15 (1995): 1917–27.

Gillman, M.W., et al. "Protective Effect of Fruits and Vegetables on Development of Stroke in Men." *Journal of the American Medical Association* 273 (1995): 1113–17.

Giovannucci, E., et al. "Multivitamin Use, Folate, and Colon Cancer in Women in the Nurses' Health Study." *Annals of Internal Medicine* 129 (1998): 517–24.

Green, D.M., et al. "Serum Potassium Level and Dietary Potassium Intake as Risk Factors for Stroke." *Neurology* 59 (2002): 314–20.

Grundy, S.M., and G.L. Vega. "Plasma Cholesterol Responsiveness to Saturated Fatty Acids." *American Journal of Clinical Nutrition* 47 (1988): 822–24.

Grundy, S.M. "What Is the Desirable Ratio of Saturated, Polyunsaturated, and Monounsaturated Fatty Acids in the Diet?" *American Journal of Clinical Nutrition* 66, suppl. (1997): 988S–990S.

Haddy, F.J., and M.B. Pamnani. "Role of Dietary Salt in Hypertension." *Journal of the American College of Nutrition* 14 (1995): 428–38.

Heart Protection Study Collaborative Group. "MRC/BHF Heart Protection Study of Antioxidant Vitamin Supplementation in 20,536 High-Risk Individuals: A Randomised Placebo-Controlled Trial." *The Lancet* 360 (2002): 23.

Hennekens, C.H., et al. "Lack of Effect of Long-Term Supplementation with Beta-Carotene on the Incidence of Malignant Neoplasms and Cardiovascular Disease." *New England Journal of Medicine* 334 (1996): 1145–49.

Hopkins, P.N. "Effects of Dietary Cholesterol on Serum Cholesterol: A Meta-Analysis and Review." *American Journal of Clinical Nutrition* 55 (1992): 1060–70.

Hu, F.B., et al. "Dietary Intake and the Risk of Coronary Heart Disease in Women." *New England Journal of Medicine.* 337 (1997): 1491–99.

Jha, P., et al. "The Antioxidant Vitamins and Cardiovascular Disease: A Critical Review of Epidemiologic and Clinical Trial Data." *Annals of Internal Medicine* 123 (1995): 860–72.

Kant, A.K., et al. "A Prospective Study of Diet Quality and Mortality in Women." *Journal of the American Medical Association* 283 (2000): 2109–15.

Knopp, R.H., et al. "Long-Term Cholesterol-Lowering Effects of Four Fat-Restricted Diets in Hypercholesterolemic and Combined Hyperlipidemic Men. The Dietary Alternatives Study." *Journal of the American Medical Association* 278 (1997): 1509–15.

Kuller, L.H. "Dietary Fat and Chronic Diseases: Epidemiologic Overview." *Journal of the American Dietary Association* 97, suppl. (1997): S9–S15.

Levinson, W., and D. Altkorn. "Primary Prevention of Postmenopausal Osteoporosis." *Journal of the American Medical Association* 280 (1998): 1821–32.

Lichtenstein, A.H., et al. "Effects of Different Forms of Dietary Hydrogenated Fats on Serum Lipoprotein Cholesterol Levels." *New England Journal of Medicine* 340 (1999): 1933–40.

Mensink, R.P., and M.B. Katan. "Effect of Dietary Fatty Acids on Serum Lipids and Lipoproteins. A Meta-Analysis of 27 Trials." *Arteriosclerosis, Thrombosis, and Vascular Biology* 12 (1992): 911–19.

NIH Consensus Development Panel on Osteoporosis Prevention, Diagnosis and Treatment. "Osteoporosis, Prevention, and Treatment." *Journal of the American Medical Association* 285 (2001): 785–95.

Nygard, O., et al. "Major Lifestyle Determinants of Plasma Total Homocysteine Distribution: The Hordaland Homocysteine Study." *American Journal of Clinical Nutrition* 67 (1998): 263–70.

Ornish, D., et al. "Can Lifestyle Changes Reverse Coronary Artery Heart Disease?" *The Lancet* 336 (1990): 129–33.

Osganian, S.K., et al. "Dietary Carotenoids and Risk of Coronary Artery Disease in Women." *American Journal of Clinical Nutrition* 77 (2003): 1390–99.

Pearson, T.A., et al. "AHA Guidelines for Primary Prevention of Cardiovascular Disease and Stroke: 2002 Update: Consensus Panel Guide to Comprehensive Risk Reduction for Adult Patients Without Coronary or Other Atherosclerotic Vascular Diseases." *Circulation* 106 (2002): 388–91.

Rimm, E.B., et al. "Folate and Vitamin B6 from Diet and Supplements in Relation to Risk of Coronary Heart Disease Among Women." *Journal of the American Medical Association* 279 (1998): 359–64.

Rimm, E.B., et al. "Vitamin E Consumption and the Risk of Coronary Heart Disease in Men." *New England Journal of Medicine* 328 (1993): 1450.

Ruxton, C.H.S., and T.R. Kirk. "Breakfast: A Review of Associations with Measures of Dietary Intake, Physiology, and Biochemistry." *British Journal of Nutrition* 78 (1997): 199–213.

Sacks, F.M., et al. "Effects on Blood Pressure of Reduced Dietary Sodium and the Dietary Approaches to Stop Hypertension (DASH) Diet." *New England Journal of Medicine* 344 (2001): 3–10.

Selhub, J., et al. "Vitamin Status and Intake as Primary Determinants of Homocysteinemia in an Elderly Population." *Journal of the American Medical Association* 270 (1993): 2693–98.

Simopoulos, A.P. "The Mediterranean Diet: What Is So Special about the Diet of Greece? The Scientific Evidence." *Journal of Nutrition* 131, suppl. (2001): 3065S–73S.

"The Sixth Report of the Joint National Committee on Prevention, Detection, Evaluation, and Treatment of High Blood Pressure." *Archives of Internal Medicine* 157 (1997): 2413–46.

Stampfer, M.J., et al. "Primary Prevention of Coronary Heart Disease in Women Through Diet and Lifestyle." *New England Journal of Medicine* 343, no. 1 (2000): 16–22.

Stampfer, M.J., et al. "Vitamin E Consumption and the Risk of Coronary Disease in Women." *New England Journal of Medicine* 328 (1993): 1444.

Todd, S., et al. "Dietary Antioxidant Vitamins and Fiber in the Etiology of Cardiovascular Disease and All-Causes Mortality: Results from the Scottish Heart Health Study." *American Journal of Epidemiology*. 150 (1999): 1073–80.

Tribble, D.L. "AHA Science Advisory—Antioxidant Consumption and Risk of Coronary Heart Disease, Emphasis on Vitamin C, Vitamin E, and Beta-Carotene: A Statement for Healthcare Professionals from the American Heart Association." *Circulation* 99 (1999): 591–95.

Trichopoulou, A., et al. "Adherence to a Mediterranean Diet and Survival in a

Greek Population." *New England Journal of Medicine* 348 (2003): 2599–2608.

van Poppel, G., et al. "Antioxidants and Coronary Heart Disease." *Annals of Medicine* 26 (1994): 429–24.

Weinberger, M.H. "Salt Sensitivity of Blood Pressure in Humans." *Hypertension* 27, part 2 (1996): 481–90.

Willett, W.C., et al. "Coffee Consumption and Coronary Heart Disease in Women: A 10-Year Follow-Up." *Journal of the American Medical Association* 275 (1996): 458–62.

Wolk, A., et al. "Long-Term Intake of Dietary Fiber and Decreased Risk of Coronary Heart Disease Among Women." *Journal of the American Medical Association* 281 (1999): 1998–2004.

Yusuf S., et al., for The Heart Outcomes Prevention Evaluation Study Investigators. "Vitamin E Supplementation and Cardiovascular Events in High-Risk Patients." *New England Journal of Medicine* 342 (2000): 154.

CHAPTER 5: EATING FOR WEIGHT CONTROL

Calle, E.E., et al. "Overweight, Obesity, and Mortality from Cancer in a Prospectively Studied Cohort of U.S. Adults." *New England Journal of Medicine* 348 (2003): 1625–38.

Despres, J.P., et al. "Hyperinsulinemia as an Independent Risk Factor for Ischemic Heart Disease." *New England Journal of Medicine* 334 (1996): 952–57.

Dorn, J.M., et al. "Body Mass Index and Mortality in a General Population Sample of Men and Women: The Buffalo Health Study." *American Journal of Epidemiology* 146 (1997): 919–31.

Eckel, R.H., and R.M. Krauss, for the AHA Nutrition Committee. "American Heart Association Call to Action: Obesity as a Major Risk Factor for Coronary Heart Disease." *Circulation* 97 (1998): 2099–2100.

Ford, E.S., et al. "Prevalence of Metabolic Syndrome Among U.S. Adults: Findings from the Third National Health and Nutrition Examination Survey." *Journal of the American Medical Association* 287 (2002): 356–59.

Klem, M.L. "Successful Losers. The Habits of Individuals Who Have Maintained Long-Term Weight Loss." *Minnesota Medicine* 83 (2000): 218–27.

Longo, V.D., and C.E. Finch. "Evolutionary Medicine: From Dwarf Model Systems to Healthy Centenarians?" *Science* 299 (2003): 1342–46.

Mokdad, A.H., et al. "The Continuing Epidemics of Obesity and Diabetes in the United States." *Journal of the American Medical Association* 286 (2001): 1195–1200.

Mokdad, A.H., et al. "Prevalence of Obesity, Diabetes, and Obesity-Related Health Risk Factors, 2001." *Journal of the American Medical Association* 289 (2003): 76–79.

National Institutes of Health, and National Heart, Lung and Blood Institute. *Clinical Guidelines on the Identification, Evaluation, and Treatment of Overweight and Obesity in Adults: The Evidence Report.* Washington, DC: U.S. Department of Health and Human Services, 1998.

Newby, P.K. "Dietary Patterns and Changes in Body Mass Index and Waist
    Circumference in Adults." *American Journal of Clinical Nutrition* 77 (2003):
    1417–25.
Taubes, G. "What If It's All Been a Big Fat Lie?" *New York Times Magazine* July 7,
    2002.
Weindruch, R. and R. Sohal. "Caloric Intake and Aging." *New England Journal of
    Medicine* 337 (1997): 986–94.

CHAPTER 6: ALCOHOL
Doll, R., et al. "Mortality in Relation to Consumption of Alcohol: 13 Years' Obser-
    vations on Male British Doctors." *British Medical Journal* 309 (1994): 911–18.
Gill, J.S, et al. "Alcohol Consumption: A Risk Factor for Hemorrhagic and Non-
    hemorrhagic Stroke." *American Journal of Medicine* 90 (1991): 489–97.
Graziano, J.M., et al. "Moderate Alcohol Intake, Increased Levels of High-Density
    Lipoprotein and Its Subfractions, and Decreased Risk of Myocardial Infarction."
    New England Journal of Medicine 329 (1993): 1829–34.
Gronbaek, M., et al. "Type of Alcohol Consumed and Mortality from All Causes,
    Coronary Heart Disease, and Cancer." *Annals of Internal Medicine* 133 (2000):
    411–19.
Klatsky, A.L. "Should Patients with Heart Disease Drink Alcohol." *Journal of the
    American Medical Association* 285 (2001): 2004–2006.
McElduff, P. and A.J. Dobson. "How Much Alcohol and How Often? Population
    Based Case-Control Study of Alcohol Consumption and Risk of a Major Coro-
    nary Event." *British Medical Journal* 314 (1997): 18–23.
Mukamai, K.J., et al. "Alcohol Consumption and Hemostatic Factors: Analysis
    of the Framingham Offspring Cohort." *Circulation* 104 (2001): 1367–73.
Muntwyler, J., et al. "Mortality and Light to Moderate Alcohol Consumption
    After Myocardial Infarction." *The Lancet* 352 (1998): 1882–85.
Rehm, J.T., et al. "Alcohol Consumption and Coronary Heart Disease Morbidity
    and Mortality." *American Journal of Epidemiology* 146 (1997): 495–501.
Renaud, S., and M. de Lorgeril. "Wine, Alcohol, Platelets, and the French Para-
    dox for Coronary Heart Disease." *The Lancet* 339 (1992): 1523–26.
Rimm, E. "Alcohol and Coronary Heart Disease: Can We Learn More?" *Epidemi-
    ology* 12 (2001): 380–82.
Rimm, E.B., et al. "Prospective Study of Alcohol Consumption and Risk of Coro-
    nary Disease in Men." *The Lancet* 338 (1991): 464–68.
Rimm, E.B., et al. "Review of Moderate Alcohol Consumtiion and Reduced Risk
    of Coronary Heart Disease: Is the Effect Due to Beer, Wine, or Spirits?" *British
    Medical Journal* 312 (1996): 731–36.
Stamper, M.J., et al. "A Prospective Study of Moderate Alcohol Consumption and
    the Risk of Coronary Disease and Stroke in Women." *New England Journal of
    Medicine.* 319 (1988): 267–73.
Thun, M.J., et al. "Alcohol Consumption and Mortality Among Middle-Aged and
    Elderly U.S. Adults." *New England Journal of Medicine* 337 (1997): 1705–14.

CHAPTER 7: SMOKING

Bazzano, L.A., et al. "Relationship Between Cigarette Smoking and Novel Risk Factors for Cardiovascular Disease in the United States." *Annals of Internal Medicine* 138 (2003): 891–99.

Benowitz, N.L., et al. "Influence of Smoking Fewer Cigarettes on Exposure to Tar, Nicotine, and Carbon Monoxide." *New England Journal of Medicine* 315 (1986): 1310–13.

Breslau, N., et al. "Nicotine Dependence in the United States: Prevalence, Trends, and Smoking Persistence." *Archives of General Psychiatry* 58 (2001): 810–16.

Cook, D.G., and D.P. Strachan "Health Effects of Passive Smoking: 3. Parental Smoking and Prevalence of Respiratory Symptoms and Asthma in School Age Children." *Thorax* 52 (1997): 1081–94.

Doll, R., et al. "Mortality in Relation to Smoking: 40 Years' Observations on Male British Doctors." *British Medical Journal* 309 (1994): 901–11.

Enstrom, J.E., and G.C. Kabat. "Environmental Tobacco Smoke and Tobacco-Related Mortality in a Prospective Study of Californians, 1960–98." *British Medical Journal.* 326 (2003): 1057–61.

Godtfredsen, N., et al. "Smoking Reduction, Smoking Cessation, and Mortality: A 16-Year Follow-Up of 19,732 Men and Women from the Copenhagen Center for Prospective Population Studies." *American Journal of Epidemiology* 156 (2001): 994–1001.

Hughes, J.R., et al. "A Meta-Analysis of the Efficacy of Over-the-Counter Nicotine Replacement." *Tobacco Control* 12 (2003): 21–27.

Hurt, R.D., et al. "A Comparison of Sustained-Release Bupropion and Placebo for Smoking Cessation." *New England Journal of Medicine* 337 (1997): 1195–1202.

Jorenby, D.E., et al. "A Controlled Trial of Sustained-Release Bupropion, a Nicotine Patch, or Both for Smoking Cessation." *New England Journal of Medicine* 340 (1999): 685–91.

Karnath, B. "Smoking Cessation." *American Journal of Medicine* 112 (2002): 399–405.

LaCroix, A.Z. "Smoking and Mortality Among Older Men and Women in Three Communities." *New England Journal of Medicine* 324 (1991): 1619–25.

Moran, S., et al. "Women Smokers' Perceptions of Smoking-Related Health Risks." *Journal of Women's Health* 12 (2003): 363–71.

Pirkle, J.L., et al. "Exposure of the U.S. Population to Environmental Tobacco Smoke: The Third National Health and Nutrition Examination Survey, 1988 to 1991." *Journal of the American Medical Association* 275 (1996): 1233–40.

Shiffman, S., et al. "Efficacy of a Nicotine Lozenge for Smoking Cessation." *Archives of Internal Medicine* 162 (2002): 1267–76.

Strachan, D.P., and D.G. Cook. "Health Effects of Passive Smoking: 6. Parental Smoking and Childhood Asthma; Longitudinal and Case-Control Studies." *Thorax* 53 (1998): 204–12.

Tashkin, D., et al. "Smoking Cessation in Patients with Chronic Obstructive Pulmonary Disease: A Double-Blind, Placebo-Controlled, Randomised Trial." *The Lancet* 357 (2002): 1571–75.

CHAPTER 8: SLEEP

D'Ambrosio, C., et al. "Quality of Life in Patients with Obstructive Sleep Apnea—
Effect of Nasal Continuous Positive Airway Pressure: A Prospective Study."
Chest 115 (1999): 123–29.

George, C.F.P., and A. Smiley. "Sleep Apnea and Automobile Crashes." *Sleep* 22
(1999): 790–95.

Gillin, J.C., and W.F. Byerley. "The Diagnosis and Management of Insomnia."
New England Journal of Medicine 322 (1990): 239–48.

Gislason, T., et al. "Snoring, Hypertension, and Sleep Apnea Syndrome: An Epi-
demiological Survey of Middle-Aged Women." *Chest* 103 (1993): 1147–51.

Holbrook, A.M., et al. "The Diagnosis and Management of Insomnia in Clinical
Practice: A Practical Evidence-Based Approach." *Canadian Medical Association
Journal* 16 (2000): 216–20.

Hu, F.B., et al. "Prospective Study of Snoring and Risk of Hypertension in
Women." *American Journal of Epidemiology* 150 (1999): 806–16.

Hu, F.B., et al. "Snoring and Risk of Cardiovascular Disease in Women." *Journal
of the American College of Cardiology* 35 (2000): 308–13.

Jennum, P., and A. Sjol. "Snoring, Sleep Apnea, and Cardiovascular Risk Factors:
The MONICA II Study." *International Journal of Epidemiology* 22 (1993): 439–44.

Kupfer, D.J., and C.F. Reynolds. "Management of Insomnia." *New England Journal of Medicine* 336 (1997): 341–46.

Loh, N.K., et al. "Do Patients with Obstructive Sleep Apnea Wake Up with
Headaches?" *Archives of Internal Medicine* 159 (1999): 1765–68.

Morin, C.M., et al. "Nonpharmacologic Treatment of Chronic Insomnia: An
American Academy of Sleep Medicine Review." *Sleep* 22 (1999): 1134–56.

Nieto, F.G., et al., for the Sleep Heart Health Study. "Association of Sleep Disordered Breathing, Sleep Apnea, and Hypertension in a Large Community-Based
Study." *Journal of the American Medical Association* 283 (2000): 1829–36.

Roth, T., and S. Ancoli-Israel. "Daytime Consequences and Correlates of Insomnia in the United States: Results of the 1991 National Sleep Foundation
Survey—II." *Sleep* 22, suppl. 2 (1999): S354–S358.

Roth, T., et al. "Public Health and Insomnia: Consensus Statement Regarding its
Status and Needs for Future Actions." *Sleep* 22, suppl. 3 (1999): 417–20.

Sateia, M.J., et al. "Evaluation of Chronic Insomnia." *Sleep* 23 (2000): 243–302.

Teran-Santos, J., et al., and the Cooperative Group Burgos-Santander. "The Association Between Sleep Apnea and the Risk of Traffic Accidents." *New England
Journal of Medicine* 340 (1999): 847–51.

Young, T., et al. "Snoring as Part of a Dose-Response Relationship between Sleep-
Disordered Breathing and Blood Pressure." *Sleep* 19, suppl. 10 (1996):
S202–S205.

Zammit, G.K. "Quality of Life in People with Insomnia." *Sleep* 22, suppl. 2 (1999):
S379–S385.

Zwillich, C.W. "Is Untreated Sleep Apnea a Factor for Chronic Hypertension?"
Journal of the American Medical Association 283 (2000): 1880–81.

CHAPTER 9: STRESS

Blumenthal, J.A., et al. "Usefulness of Psychosocial Treatment of Mental Stress-Induced Myocardial Ischemia in Men." *American Journal of Cardiology* 89 (2002): 164–68.

Chang, P.P., et al. "Anger in Young Men and Subsequent Premature Cardiovascular Disease." *Archives of Internal Medicine* 162 (2002): 901–906.

Chaput, L.A., et al. "Hostility Predicts Recurrent Events Among Postmenopausal Women with Coronary Heart Disease." *American Journal of Epidemiology* 156 (2002): 1092–99.

Denolett, J., et al. "Personality as an Independent Predictor of Long-Term Mortality in Patients with Coronary Heart Disease." *The Lancet* 347 (1996): 417–21.

Eng, P.M., et al. "Anger Expression and Risk of Stroke and Coronary Heart Disease Among Male Health Professionals." *Psychosomatic Medicine* 65 (2003): 100–10.

Everson, S.A., et al. "Interaction of Workplace Demands and Cardiovascular Reactivity in Progression of Carotid Atheroscelrosis: Population-Based Study." *British Medical Journal* 314 (1997): 553–58.

Ginzburg, K., et al. "Repressive Coping Style, Acute Stress Disorder, and Posttraumatic Stress Disorder after Myocardial Infarction." *Psychosomatic Medicine* 64 (2002): 748–57.

Goodwin, P.J., et al. "The Effect of Group Psychosocial Support on Survival in Metastatic Breast Cancer." *New England Journal of Medicine* 345 (2001): 1719–26.

Holroyd, K.A., et al. "Management of Chronic Tension-Type Headache with Tricyclic Antidepressant Medication, Stress Management Therapy, and their Combination: A Randomized Controlled Trial." *Journal of the American Medical Association* 285 (2001): 2208–15.

Houston, B.K., et al. "Social Dominance and 22-Year All-Cause Mortality in Men." *Psychosomatic Medicine* 59 (1997): 51–57.

Kiecolt-Glaser, J.K., et al. "Marital Conflict in Older Adults: Endocrinological and Immunological Correlates." *Psychosomatic Medicine* 59 (1997): 339–49.

Kowalski, M., et al. "A New Pattern of Cardiac Events Emerges Following the World Trade Center Attack." *Circulation* 106, abstract 3710 (2002): II–755.

Macleod, J., et al. "Marital Stress and Coronary Heart Disease." *Journal of the American Medical Association* 285 (2001): 1289–90.

Marmot, M.G., et al. "Contribution of Job Control and Other Risk Factors to Social Variations in Coronary Heart Incidence." *The Lancet* 350 (1997): 235–39.

May, M., et al. "Does Psychological Distress Predict the Risk of Ischemic Stroke and Transient Ischemic Attack? The Caerphilly Study." *Stroke* 33 (2002): 7–12.

McEwen, B.S. "Protective and Damaging Effects of Stress Mediators." *New England Journal of Medicine* 338 (1998): 171–79.

Redd, W.H., et al. "Behavioral Intervention for Cancer Treatment Side Effects." *Journal of the National Cancer Institute* 93 (2001): 810–23.

Rozanski, A., et al. "Impact of Psychological Factors on the Pathogenesis of Cardiovascular Disease and Implications for Therapy." *Circulation* 99 (1999): 2192–217.

Russke, L.G., and G.E. Schwartz. "Feelings of Parental Caring Predict Health Status in Midlife: A 35-Year Follow-Up of the Harvard Mastery of Stress Study." *Journal of Behavioral Medicine* 201 (1997): 1–13.

Salovey, P., et al. "Emotional States and Physical Health." *American Psychologist* 55 (2000): 110–21.

Starkman, M.N., et al. "Elevated Cortisol Levels in Cushing's Disease Are Associated with Cognitive Decrements." *Psychosomatic Medicine* 63 (2001): 985–93.

Yan, L.L., et al. "Time Urgency/Impatience (TUI) Predicts Incident Hypertension 13 Years Later: Abstracts from American Heart Association Scientific Sessions 2002, November 17–20, 2002, Chicago, Illinois." *Circulation* 106, suppl. II (2002): II–755.

CHAPTER 10: SEX

Diokno, A.C., et al. "Sexual Function in the Elderly." *Archives of Internal Medicine* 150 (1990): 197–200.

Feldman, H.A., et al. "Impotence and Its Medical and Psychosocial Correlates: Results of the Massachusetts Male Aging Study." *Journal of Urology* 151 (1994): 54–61.

Jacoby, S. "Great Sex: What's Age Got to Do With It?" *Modern Maturity*, Sept.–Oct. 1999.

Laumann, E.O., et al. "Sexual Dysfunction in the United States: Prevalence and Predictors." *Journal of the American Medical Association* 281 (1999): 537–44.

Muller, J., et al. "Triggering Myocardial Infarction by Sexual Activity." *Journal of the American Medical Association* 275 (1996): 1405–9.

Thienhaus, O.J. "Practical Overview of Sexual Function and Advancing Age. *Geriatrics* 43 (1988): 63–67.

Wiley, D., and W.M. Bortz, II. "Sexuality and Aging: Usual and Successful." *Journal of Gerontology* 51A (1996): M142–M146.

CHAPTER 11: ISSUES TO DISCUSS WITH YOUR DOCTOR

American Diabetes Association. "Aspirin Therapy in Diabetes." *Diabetes Care* 20 (1997): 1772–73.

Antithrombotic Trialists' Collaboration. "Collaborative Meta-Analysis of Randomised Trials of Antiplatelet Therapy for Prevention of Death, Myocardial Infarction, and Stroke in High-Risk Patients." *British Medical Journal* 324 (2002): 71–86.

Antiplatelet Trialists' Collaboration. "Collaborative Overview of Randomized Trials of Antiplatelet Therapy. I: Prevention of Death, Myocardial Infarction, and Stroke by Prolonged Antiplatelet Therapy in Various Categories of Patients." *British Medical Journal* 308 (1994): 81–106.

Baron, J.A., et al. "A Randomized Trial of Aspirin to Prevent Colorectal Adenomas." *New England Journal of Medicine* 348 (2003): 891–99.

Baxter, N. "Preventive Health Care 2001 Update: Should Women Be Routinely Taught Breast Self-Examination to Screen for Breast Cancer?" *Canadian Medical Association Journal* 164 (2001): 1837–46.

Cadarette, S.M., et al. "Evaluation of Decision Rules for Referring Women for Bone Densitometry by Dual-Energy X-Ray Absorptiometry." *Journal of the American Medical Association* 286 (2001): 57–63.

Centers for Disease Control and Prevention. *Sexually Transmitted Diseases Treatment Guidelines: 2002.* Atlanta, GA: U.S. Department of Health and Human Services, 2002. MMWR 2002; 51(RR-6): 2.

Dabaghi, S.F., et al. "Effects of Low-Dose Aspirin on In Vitro Platelet Aggregation in the Early Minutes after Ingestion in Normal Subjects." *American Journal of Cardiology* 74 (1994): 720–23.

Davis, C.E., et al. "A Single Cholesterol Measurement Underestimates the Risk of Coronary Heart Disease: An Empirical Example from the Lipid Research Clinics Mortality Follow-Up Study." *Journal of the American Medical Association* 264 (1990): 3044–46.

Duffy, S.W., et al. "The Impact of Organized Mammography Service Screening on Breast Carcinoma Mortality in Seven Swedish Counties." *Cancer* 94 (2002): 458–69.

Engelgau, M.E., et al. "Screening for Type 2 Diabetes." *Diabetes Care* 10 (2000): 1563–80.

Expert Panel On Detection, Evaluation, and Treatment of High Blood Cholesterol in Adults. "Executive Summary of the Third Report of the National Cholesterol Education Program (NCEP) Expert Panel on Detection, Evaluation, and Treatment of High Blood Cholesterol in Adults (Adult Treatment Panel III)." *Journal of the American Medical Association* 285 (2001): 2486–97.

Ferrini, R., and S.H. Woolf. "American College of Preventive Medicine Practice Policy: Screening for Prostate Cancer in American Men." *American Journal of Preventive Medicine* 15 (1998): 81–84.

Gan, S.C., et al. "Treatment of Acute Myocardial Infarction and 30-Day Mortality Among Women and Men." *New England Journal of Medicine* 343 (2000): 8–15.

Gotzsche, P.C., and O. Olsen. "Is Screening for Breast Cancer with Mammography Justifiable?" *The Lancet* 355 (2000): 129–34.

Gum, P.A., et al. "Aspirin and All-Cause Mortality Among Patients Being Evaluated for Known or Suspected Coronary Artery Disease: A Propensity Analysis." *Journal of the American Medical Association* 286 (2001): 1187–94.

Hak, A.E., et al. "Subclinical Hypothyroidism Is an Independent Risk Factor for Atherosclerosis and Myocardial Infarction in Elderly Women: The Rotterdam Study." *Annals of Internal Medicine* 132 (2000): 270–78.

Hansson, L., et al. "Effects of Intensive Blood-Pressure Lowering and Low-Dose Aspirin in Patients with Hypertension: Principal Results of the Hypertension Optimal Treatment (HOT) Randomized Trial." *The Lancet* 351 (1998): 1755–62.

Harris, R. "What Is the Right Cancer Screening Rate?" *Annals of Internal Medicine* 132 (2000): 732–34.

Hayden, M., et al. "Aspirin for the Primary Prevention of Cardiovascular Events: A Summary of the Evidence for the U.S. Preventive Services Task Force." *Annals of Internal Medicine* 136 (2002): 161–72.

Krumholz, H.M., et al. "Aspirin in the Treatment of Acute Myocardial Infarction in Elderly Medicare Beneficiaries: Patterns of Use and Outcomes." *Circulation* 92 (1995): 2841–47.

Lagrand, W.K., et al. "C-Reactive Protein as a Cardiovascular Risk Factor: More Than an Epiphenomenon?" *Circulation* 100 (1999): 96–102.

Lauer, M.S. "Aspirin for Primary Prevention of Coronary Events." *New England Journal of Medicine* 346 (2002): 1468–74.

Mandelblatt, J.S., and K.R. Yabroff. "Breast and Cervical Cancer Screening for Older Women: Recommendations and Challenges for the 21st Century." *Journal of the American Medical Women's Association* 55 (2000): 210–15.

McGovern, P.G., et al. "Recent Trends in Acute Coronary Heart Disease—Mortality, Morbidity, Medical Care, and Risk Factors." *New England Journal of Medicine* 334 (1996): 884–90.

North American Menopause Society. "Management of Postmenopausal Osteoporosis: Position Statement of the North American Menopause Society." *Menopause* 9 (2002): 84–101.

Olsen, O., and P.C. Gotzsche. "Cochrane Review on Screening for Breast Cancer with Mammography." *The Lancet* 358 (2001): 1340–42.

Pignone, M.P., et al. "Screening and Treating Adults for Lipid Disorders." *American Journal of Preventive Medicine* 20, suppl. 3 (2001): 77–89.

Ridker, P.M., et al. "Inflammation, Aspirin, and the Risk of Cardiovascular Disease in Apparently Healthy Men." *New England Journal of Medicine* 336 (1997): 973–76.

Ridker, P.M., et al. "Novel Risk Factors for Systemic Atherosclerosis: A Comparison of C-Reactive Protein, Fibrinogen, Homocysteine, Lipoprotein(a), and Standard Cholesterol Screening as Predictors of Peripheral Arterial Disease." *Journal of the American Medical Association* 285 (2001): 2481–85.

Solomon, D.H., et al. "Nonsteroidal Anti-Inflammatory Drug Use and Acute Myocardial Infarction." *Archives of Internal Medicine* 162 (2002): 1099–104.

Spann, S.J. "Prostate Cancer Screening—What's a Physician To Do?" *American Family Physician* 56 (1997): 1563–64, 1567–68.

Steering Committee of the Physicians' Health Study Research Group. "Final Report on the Aspirin Component of the Ongoing Physicians' Health Study." *New England Journal of Medicine* 321 (1989): 129–35.

Swan, J., et al. "Progress in Cancer-Screening Practices in the United States: Results from the 2000 National Health Interview Survey." *Cancer* 97 (2003): 1528–40.

Tabar, L., et al. "Beyond Randomized Controlled Trials: Organized Mammographic Screening Reduces Breast Carcinoma Mortality." *Cancer* 91 (2001): 1724–31.

U.S. Preventive Services Task Force. *Guide to Clinical Preventive Services, Third Edition, 2000–2003.* Washington, DC: U.S. Department of Health and Human Services, 2003. Available at: http: //www.ahcpr.gov/clinic/cps3dix.htm.

U.S. Preventive Services Task Force. "Screening for Colorectal Cancer: Recommendation and Rationale." *Annals of Internal Medicine* 137 (2002): 129–31.

Weil, J., et al. "Prophylactic Aspirin and Risk of Peptic Ulcer Bleeding." *British Medical Journal* 310 (1995): 827–30.

Winawer, S., et al. "Colorectal Cancer Screening and Surveillance: Clinical Guidelines and Rationale — Update Based on New Evidence." *Gastroenterology* 124 (2003): 544–60.

Winawer, S.J., et al. "Prevention of Colorectal Cancer by Colonoscopic Polypectomy." *New England Journal of Medicine* 329 (1993): 1977–81.

Index